D1081847

Breathless

A Transplant Surgeon's Journal

"You take giant steps over the little red line your teachers and mentors said you weren't supposed to step over. As long as I can predict there is a reasonable possibility that at the end of this I can have a viable functioning patient, then it is no holds barred. You go 4 plus all the way."

Thomas R.J. Todd, MD FRCSC

Published by

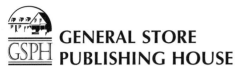

**GENERAL STORE
PUBLISHING HOUSE**

499 O'Brien Rd., Box 415, Renfrew, Ontario, Canada K7V 4A6
Telephone (613) 432-7697 or 1-800-465-6072
www.gsph.com

ISBN-13: 978-1-897113-54-7
Printed and bound in Canada

Cover design, formatting and printing by
Custom Printers of Renfrew Ltd.

No part of this book may be reproduced, stored in a retrieval system or
transmitted in any form or by any means, without the prior written permission
of the publisher or, in case of photocopying or other reprographic copying, a
licence from Access Copyright (Canadian Copyright Licensing Agency),
1 Yonge Street, Suite 1900, Toronto, Ontario, M5E 1E5.

Library and Archives Canada Cataloguing in Publication

Todd, Thomas, 1945-
    Breathless / Thomas Todd.

Includes bibliographical references.
ISBN 978-1-897113-54-7

    1. Lungs--Transplantation--Canada--History. 2. Todd, Thomas, 1945-
3. Surgeons--Canada--Biography. I. Title.

RD539.T63 2007   617.5'420592   C2007-900207-2

Dedication

To Lesley, for without her constant support,
none of this could have happened.

Acknowledgements

As a first time author, there are a host of people deserving of my thanks. Without them, what follows would never have been published. Elias Petras whose film "The Breath of Life" documented our early days kindly consented to our use of the film's scenes on the cover. Fran and bill Bawdin provided much needed direction and advice. Tim Gordon, my publisher, and Jane Karchmar, my editor have my enduring gratitude for their faith and patience. My greatest appreciation must be reserved for my son, Jeffrey, who constantly cajoled and encouraged me; and of course my wife, Lesley for her never ending confidence and support during the long years of surgical practice. I could never have done this without her encouragement, criticism and her endless hours of proof reading. But most of all I thank my father Collin who provided the spark.

Foreword

As a patient, I was aware that medical science is in a constant state of flux with advancements occurring on an almost daily basis. However, I had never had an opportunity to observe and learn the details of the commitment, the excitement, and the frustration of the process and the real people who achieve these gains.

When I became the CEO of the largest provincial medical association in Canada, the Ontario Medical Association (OMA), I discovered that I had a unique window on the personnel and processes of the practice of medicine in its clinical, political, and research dimensions. My role in the OMA, together with my friendship with the author since medical school days at Queen's University, gave me a double window on one such medical breakthrough in which the author was a principal surgeon.

Above all else, this is a story about people. It is also about the human spirit. It will impact readers whether they are medical professionals or non-professionals simply interested in a dramatic human drama about hope. We learn about the intense personal perspective of the patient and the life-and-death friendships that develop between the physician and the patient in a transplant scenario. The overwhelming sense of commitment on the part of the physicians borders on almost intolerable personal stress levels. Nowhere could there be a more sincere demonstration of the Hippocratic Oath in modern practice than the commitment of the physician colleagues who dedicate their personal and professional lives to the welfare of their transplant patients. Of course, the intensity of patient concern could not be greater than in a transplant context where success means life and failure could mean end of life

This story exposes us to the intimate details of scientific progress, some of which we may not anticipate without this kind of "insider" information—in particular, the personal energy, creativity, innovation, and team spirit of the surgical team that developed revolutionary transplant outcomes. I observed a transplant procedure that took all night between two operating rooms. The human impact of the awareness that one life was ending and another life benefiting was almost impossible to accept that evening. The emotional highs when a donor is identified, the critical nature of timing, and the emotional downs experienced by both the patient and the surgeon when cancellations occur, are all part of this human drama.

What may be more surprising is the extent to which the health care system is revealed as both an enabler and an obstacle to such innovation, with its emphasis on limited resources, restrictive policies, and the ubiquitous inertia of bureaucracy. Struggling within these system-imposed confines, the surgeons are forced to use their creative and innovative skills to achieve outcomes they know are fundamental to the lives of their patients.

My comments would not be complete without a personal note. When I had finished reading this story, I had a sense of déjà vu in that I was reminded that the medical student I knew at university and the senior surgeon who is the author of this book are the same person. Dr. Todd was a bright and committed student who simply matured into an innovative and dedicated surgeon.

David Pattenden, PhD
Past CEO, Ontario Medical Association

Prologue

It has been twenty-three years since a group of young surgeons at Toronto General Hospital performed the world's first successful lung transplant. I was fortunate to be in their number and witnessed events that were sufficiently dramatic to rival any episode of television medical programming. There were those that from the personal point of view were profoundly moving; there were others where the excitement was electric; and still others when triumph was snatched from our grasp to be replaced by dismay and self-condemnation.

Nonetheless, I recall situations that when viewed today through the eyes of retrospect are amusing, if not comical. There are so many stories locked in my head for the telling that I fret the passage of time will lead to their loss from memory or at the least become less accurate and vigorous. As I age, I recognize that such is a reality.

I recall a patient; his name was Terry, but I no longer remember his last name. I do remember that he came from Western Canada and that he required a heart-lung transplant for (I think) cystic fibrosis. Although I remain uncertain about the diagnosis, I do recall the evening when one of my Intensive Care Unit (ICU) nurses walked out of his room. It was just before his transplant. He had proposed marriage to her. She was so affected by the circumstance that she was tempted to run back in and immediately accept, despite her realization that the entire event was triggered and sustained by the emotion of the moment. Her enthusiasm would pass with the morning. I recall sitting at the nursing station as she related the story to me and thinking that for Terry this must be like the day before combat for young soldiers who know that this may be the last chance they have to experience the emotion of life. I also recall that Terry received his transplant, yet what happened thereafter is misty. He did not do well, if memory serves me, and died from either complications or rejection or both. What follows in these pages is more precise.

It was a privileged time for me, a period of great excitement, the anticipation of accomplishment, and the fulfillment of a dream. It seems a shame to let the years dull our memory and to not take the opportunity to tell the tale the way it actually happened. I know that if I don't put my recollections to pen now, the magic of the moment will be lost. Fortunately, I kept a log of the significant events. The rest is from my memory of the events themselves.

I expect that what I really want to achieve is to amuse you with the humanness of a uniquely Canadian accomplishment. And indeed it is the human side of the lung transplant story that I wish to emphasize. The technical and scientific aspects of what we accomplished were covered in detail long ago in the press and in medical journals. But there were personal things that we never discussed. Some could be misconstrued as error. Some were outlandish and for obvious reasons were never discussed in public. Other events were simply sad. They occurred and were just placed in the back reaches of our minds. It was not deemed professional to discuss them at the time. Probably that was correct. With the passage of the years, however, their telling is of less significance than it would have been then.

As it is now almost twenty-four years since the first successful transplant recipient left hospital, the operation and the entire process seem routine. Well, not quite routine— the hours are still long and the procedure itself can still be difficult and demanding. But the sense of excitement, the "stir" is gone. True, there are moments when a medical student or a surgical resident witnesses the event for the first time, and in their enthusiasm they carry you back to the feelings of the early days. Nonetheless, at some point, for me at least, it began to feel more like work. It was never that way at the beginning. Perhaps it is much like the aging athlete where accomplishment is still novel and fresh and each day brings the challenge that you may actually surpass what you did the day before. But the day comes when hitting the ball or running the track is just part of what you have to do to earn your living. As you will see in these pages, the appreciation of drama and enthusiasm waxed and waned with the sense of innovation and change. As the medical system in Canada began to be restrictive, so, too, did the feeling of individual accomplishment and the satisfaction attendant upon it.

The personal factor seems lost as well. In the first days of the Toronto Lung Transplant Program, I knew all the potential recipients intimately. Their medical histories could be recited at will, including all their laboratory data. All their important information that might play a role in the selection of a donor or in their post-operative care was firmly lodged in my memory banks. But the knowledge of the patients then went much deeper than just the medical facts of their case. I knew them as individuals. They were real people to me. I saw them frequently; each name had a face, a mother, father, or spouse. I shared their concerns and felt the tension and anticipation that dwelt in each of them. They were each unique, but were all in Toronto for one reason. This was the place to get a lung transplant. Each hoped they would secure the right donor and that one would be the first to turn history around and set the standard for the new era of pulmonary replacement. Surviving the surgery was not a given even after the first success became widely known. The prospect of imminent death amidst the fight to stay alive created a bond between surgeon and patient that in my experience remains unique.

By 1996 things were different. Then we arrive in the operating room to do a transplant often never having seen the recipient before. He/she is purely "medical information." A condition lies there on the table possessing a series of data points that I need to comprehend to ensure proper donor selection and to perform the procedure correctly.

These recipients could be anybody. I might have passed them in the halls of the hospital or ridden on the elevator with them and not known who they were, let alone understand what made them the unique people they are. Their families are strangers when I walk into the waiting room to give the good or at times the bad news. It's hard to prepare to do the job properly when you don't know who or what to expect when you walk through the doors of the waiting room. I remember the day I had to inform a family that the procedure had gone badly; that the twenty-three-year-old patient would at best suffer permanent brain damage even if she survived. As I came off the elevator and walked down the corridor, I wondered who would be waiting on the other side of the doors—husband, parents, hopefully not children. They are all still unique, still committed to the program but I no longer know them that way; and because of that, at the end of my tenure in Toronto I didn't feel the same sense of completeness that should have been present for someone who does what I did. The patients deserve better.

How did this happen? How did we lose that personal feeling, that oneness with our patients? In a word— success. Toronto General Hospital became famous overnight. We were the only ones who had successfully achieved a lung transplant. The administration opened the doors to patients from all over North America. Indeed, in the first few years of the program, there were not many Canadians on the waiting lists.

Although other programs commenced activity all over the world, it took some time before they were operational. We continued to grow. Unfortunately, our resource base grew very little. By 1996, we were undertaking fifteen times the number of transplants as the meagre three in 1985 but with fewer staff. As a result, the involvement of the surgeons in the pre-operative evaluation and preparation phases had to decrease. There were those who replaced us and they did as well as, if not better than, we did in this assessment. There was, however, something missing. The patients still wanted to relate to the surgeons who would undertake the procedure, and we certainly longed for the days when we could afford the time to hear their concerns, to discuss the event at length with them, and to get to know their fears. How else could you be the dragon slayer that each surgeon sets himself or herself out to be? How else to satisfy egos as big as the sky if you were now merely the technician—the mechanic?

I still feel a strong link to those early patients, the ones who survived and the ones who are long since gone. They were the first, and I grew to respect them and I still cherish their memory. It is for their memory and the memory of the families who consented to have their loved ones serve as donors that I wish to relate this story. It's a true story, and I have attempted to tell it as factually as possible. What follows comes from the contemporaneous notes that I took during the course of events, from my memory, and in some cases from recorded interviews with patients. The dialogue, where present, is reconstructed from my memory and, although not literal, represents an accurate recollection. I hope that you will feel their sense of anticipation, share their concerns and pain, and as well feel the dismay of defeat. These folks whose lives were destined to be short truly loved the life they had to the fullest. We can learn from them. I did. I hope you can, too.

CHAPTER 1

The Beginning

A spring day in Toronto is truly to be savoured. Blue skies and moderate temperatures predominate and the sun shines reliably. In the downtown core along "hospital row" south of Queen's Park, the seat of the Ontario government, the arrival of the warmth is particularly appreciated. The flower beds along University Avenue leading up to the legislative buildings are vibrantly in full bloom. People have reclaimed the sidewalks. The cafés and even the hospital coffee shops have laid their own claim to the concrete with their plastic tables and chairs. The hospital and office workers purchase their lunches from the ubiquitous fast-food hawkers under their brightly coloured umbrellas and then lounge on the benches that perch on the few islands of greenery. The civil servants sprawl on the more substantial legislative lawns. Doctors and nurses in scrub suits and white lab coats dodge the traffic as they run between Toronto General, Mt. Sinai, and the Hospital for Sick Children. Groups of businessmen smartly outfitted in the best that Nike can offer pad down the sidewalk avoiding the walkers by stepping out onto the street, while the business ladies jogging in their spandex suits part the crowd like a ripple on a pond. After a long and dreary winter, the city has come to life. It's a wonderful time in a truly great metropolis.

University Avenue is without doubt the showpiece of the downtown core. With the Waterfront and Queen's Quay at one end and the dominating façade of the legislative building at the other, it cuts through the heart of the city. It is lined with tall, glass office complexes, consulates, hotels, and most particularly with hospitals—five in number, four of which flank the top of the street below the legislature.

The world-famous Sick Children's Hospital is an old brownstone building whose age is belied by the glass atrium of the modern addition that faces Elizabeth street just east of University Avenue. The addition's atrium is festooned with balconies and catwalks. Its presentation to the street announces to all that it is a place for the little ones with its meagre lawn arrayed with statues of animals and a wonderful modern brass sculpture of a mother holding her ailing child.

Across the street is the old Mount Sinai Hospital, now a rehabilitation facility bearing the name of England's second Elizabeth. It is a dowdy yellow, clearly aging and unkempt twelve-storey building, its condition a mighty reflection of the regard Canadian society places on the rehabilitation of its chronically afflicted. Beside it, however, is the grey stone elegant edifice of the new eighteen-storey Mount Sinai, which, although it was constructed in the 1970s, still looks young and fresh compared to its counterparts on University Avenue. It blends nicely with the neoclassical architecture of the Princess Margaret Hospital next door. The latter is a beautiful restoration of the façade of a century-old bank building complete with Corinthian columns and an ornately carved balustrade. Behind the façade, the building is all new, complete with the atrium and catwalks that characterized so much of hospital construction in the latter part of the century. It is light and airy inside, whereas the façade provides the sense of security and permanence of the last century—a great combination for a hospital that has dedicated itself to the care of cancer patients.

Across the street from the new Mount Sinai and sprawling across an entire city block is Canada's oldest academic hospital. A conglomerate of towers, both modern and by Canadian standards ancient (i.e. just over a hundred years old), it hardly appears as a single structure but rather a city unto itself. To generations of physicians and patients, it was known as The Toronto General Hospital. But in the late 1980s hospital restructuring came to Canada. The "big house," as it was known to my generation, underwent a bureaucratically driven metamorphosis. It became the Toronto Hospital when a merger was fashioned with the Toronto Western Hospital.

"Merger" was indeed a euphemism for downsizing and a general reduction in health care delivery. In fact, it took a formal piece of legislation in the province of Ontario to create the new designation. Within a decade it would change its name again, following yet another merger with the Princess Margaret Hospital. This time it underwent a formal "branding" process, which lasted several months at an incredible cost. It seems that some consultant or other determined that branding was the essential ingredient of subsequent success. Names such as the Upper Canada Hospital and the Great Lakes Hospital Association were considered. These sounded much like a bakery or a brewery to most of us, but indeed they were on the official list of suggestions. After much publicity and a reportedly hefty profit for the consultant, a novel name was developed: why, we would become the Toronto General Hospital of the University Health Network. How unique!

At any rate, we retrieved the "General"; the term "University Health Network," despite all the fanfare of new stationery and logos, would be merely something that still lurked in the minds of our self-important administrative staff. All the name changes could not impact on the mystique of this place. It is the hub of Canadian medicine. Here, Banting discovered insulin; the first renal dialysis was conducted; heparin was discovered; Wilfred Bigelow developed the concept of hypothermia, which was to revolutionize cardiac surgery.

But beyond the innovations, it was a place of the supreme clinician and surgeon. It was known for "going beyond." The stories of our forebears—their quirks, their foibles, and their passion—was the stuff of legend. I avoided it like the plague during my first years of surgical training. The entire atmosphere was said to be intimidating and oblivious to the personal needs of patients and surgical residents alike. The rumour mill in the residency circles was simply that careers could well be shaped and established here, but they were likewise frequently destroyed. Here you had to be good to survive.

Hospitals are sombre places, but spring is a happy time there, too. The courtyards, sidewalks, and entranceways are lined with wheelchairs and patients pushing rickety IV poles, wearing a mixture of hospital and street garb. Despite sickness and pain, the patients appeared cheered by the signs of summer's coming. Of course for many, the cheer comes directly from the stimulant effect of the tobacco that they have longed for during their time in the smoke-free environment of the hospital. Despite that, there is an emotional warmth that comes from the feel of the sun on your face, and a not too unrealistic belief that such can only speed the healing process that the physicians have hopefully initiated. Even here there is a sense of rebirth, of healing, of getting well again. For most, but not for all.

I have a picture in my academic slide collection of a seventeen-year-old boy out on the lawn of the hospital; lawn that has since fallen victim to the hospital's relentless expansion. Today it's a driveway into the Eaton Wing. The boy has a tracheostomy in place and looks frail and wan. His hair is dishevelled and he is attired in the standard hospital blue gown that has slipped off one shoulder; his spindly legs capped off with paper slippers are poking out from the gown's irregular hem. A nurse holds an IV bag over the boy's head and if one strains the eye, the plastic tubing snaking downwards to his arm becomes visible. His entire habitus looks strained and tired. But he is smiling—a glorious full smile—despite the circumstances. For today is his birthday and he is alive. Not only alive, but actually outside his hospital room after months of confinement in an ICU bed following a severe inhalation burn that destroyed his lungs. He holds on to and is in part supported by the bicycle given to him by his parents to commemorate much more than just his birthday. It is 1977. I never knew the boy, but I see his face so often when I think of how it all began—for in truth, it began with him. Seventeen days previously, he had become the thirty-ninth person in history to receive a single lung transplant.

He was about to become as well the thirty-ninth fatality. Two days after his picture was taken on the lawn of Toronto General Hospital, he was once again in the operating room. After several hours of surgery, the hopes of his family and the aspirations of the surgical team would be dealt a lethal blow.

A lung has three connections to the rest of your body (please see Glossary for following terminology). The first is the air tube or bronchus that joins to your main air tube or trachea that you can feel in your neck. The second is the pulmonary artery that brings blood to the lungs to receive oxygen; and the third are the pulmonary veins (two per lung) that return blood now rich in oxygen to the heart for distribution to the rest of your body.

In this young man's case, the surgically created communication (called an anastomosis) between the donor air tube (bronchus) and his own air tube had come apart. Although the surgeons knew that the chances of correcting the problem were remote, the attempt had to be made. He was rushed back to the operating room. He would not survive.

The breakdown of the suture line between the donor and recipient air tubes (the bronchial anastomosis) was the Achilles heel of lung transplantation for reasons I will make clear later. Most of the previous forty failures had been a result of this complication. This patient was about to become another statistic,

THOMAS R.J. TODD, MD FRCSC | **5**

another failure to add to the growing list. But in the death of this young man there was to be a difference. Although he was the thirty-ninth person to undergo a single lung transplant, he was the first one to have the procedure undertaken at Toronto General. The difference lay in an unwillingness to accept defeat and in the belief that nothing was impossible—one simply had to learn from the failure by an analysis of the chain of events and by improvisation designed to permanently correct the problem.

This principle guided the nature of the observations made that day in the midst of defeat and despair for the family and the medical team. It was the combination of intense, unemotional observation with a determination to succeed that would initiate the events of the next six years. Ten people can observe the same event, but only one might see the entirety of it all. Some never see beyond the visual expression; others see and understand the complexities that lay behind casual observation. It was to be that way in this case.

While the rest of the team noted that his demise had been secondary to the disruption of his bronchial anastomosis, one surgeon noted that the healing of the other connections (the artery and the veins) between the donor lung and the patient, although intact, were also fragile and showing early signs of disruption. *Could it be that the failure to heal was a generalized phenomenon not unique to the airway, but expressed here first because the bronchus was the most susceptible?*

Prior to that day, it was assumed that the connection between the donor bronchus and that of the recipient was prone to poor healing because of either rejection, inadequate blood supply, or both. Whatever the cause, it was considered to be a problem unique to that anatomical site. The observations that day, however, suddenly placed a new question on the table. Could it be that there is a generalized problem with healing in these individuals? As with so many advances in science, to find the right answers one must first ask the correct questions.

I have often wished that I had been there at that moment and to have been a part of the discussion and analysis that would lead ultimately to success. Although I would participate in the exciting times to come, my involvement was yet to become a reality. Yet I begrudge my absence that day, for that's the most important part—when the idea is fresh and the excitement palpable.

In 1977, I was beginning my practice at Queen's University in Kingston, having left Toronto General the year before at the completion of my Thoracic Surgical training. My teachers performed the transplant on this young man and asked the right questions at the end of it all. I watched enviously from afar. My only involvement was to send a sample of blood by military aircraft to Toronto for tissue typing from a brain-dead patient at Kingston General Hospital in the hope that he might serve as the donor for this young man. The plane took off into a pelting rainstorm as I watched from my car beside the tiny Kingston airstrip. The donor, however, was not a proper match, and I was to hear of Toronto's first attempt at lung transplantation after the fact. Nine years later, I would again be in Kingston, in another violent storm, this time arriving in a Lear Jet to extract the donor lungs for the world's first successful double lung transplant. But in 1977, it appeared that the transplantation of a lung was impossible.

Before we proceed further to chronicle the events, we first need to spend some technical time on the medical aspects of lung (or pulmonary) transplantation, so that the reader can better appreciate what is to follow. Dr. James Hardy performed the first attempt at lung transplantation in 1963 in Mississippi. Several others followed as the interest in transplantation of all sorts blossomed in the '60s and '70s. They all failed. Kidney transplantation was a fact before I entered medical school. Heart transplantation became a reality before I graduated, although its acceptance by a too-eager and too-enthusiastic surgical community led to significant problems for the next several years. The failure of lung transplantation prior to 1983 was in retrospect the result of a multitude of unrelated factors. Indeed, even after the first success in 1983, we still failed to appreciate the constellation of factors that in reality reversed the tide of the preceding twenty years.

But I am ahead of myself. It is important to appreciate the state of the art in 1978 and the concepts we had of why failure was the ubiquitous result of attempts to transplant a lung. To fully understand the reasons behind this and the stories of the early patients that follow, it is necessary to know how the lung functions and how a transplant is performed. Thus what follows is a bit of physiology that I promise will be brief.

It's all about oxygen and how it gets to the tissues of your body. Without it, our cells and the organs they make up cannot perform. The lung exchanges oxygen and carbon dioxide between your bloodstream and the air that you breathe. You inhale oxygen-rich air, which contains virtually no carbon dioxide. Your heart pumps blood low in oxygen and high in carbon dioxide to the lung after the blood has been through your tissues where the oxygen is extracted to provide fuel for your metabolism. The carbon dioxide is added at the tissue level as a product of that metabolism.

Your heart has two sides that enable the appropriate separation of blood rich in oxygen from that portion where the oxygen levels are low. Figure 1 attempts to schematically represent the anatomy and blood flow of the heart. For simplicity's sake the figure represents the heart as a single chamber, whereas in fact there are two sides as noted above. The blood poor in oxygen and rich in carbon dioxide arrives in the right side of the heart from the body tissues via the extensive system of veins culminating in the superior and inferior vena cava. It first enters the right atrium and then is propelled through a valve into the right ventricle, which contracts to push the blood to the lungs via the pulmonary arteries. Each pulmonary artery divides progressively into smaller and smaller vessels; the ones that surround the tiny terminal air sacs in your lungs are microscopic and have extremely thin and porous walls.

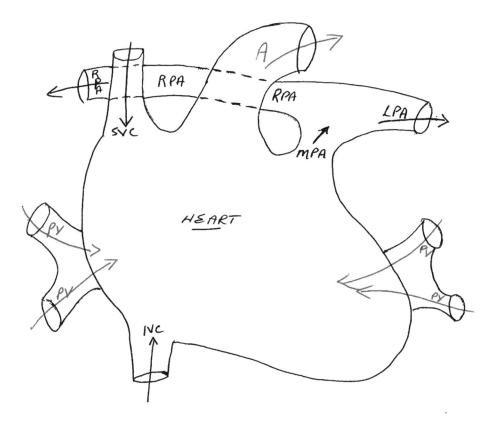

A = aorta; RPA = right pulmonary artery; MPA = main pulmonary artery;
LPA = left pulmonary artery; SVC =superior vena cava;
IVC = inferior vena cava; PV = pulmonary vein

Figure 1. Diagram of the heart and great vessels.

It is here at the microscopic level that the blood absorbs oxygen from the air sacs and gives up carbon dioxide through this thin, porous membrane. The exchange takes place because the concentration of the two gases across the membrane is different. With each breath you take, carbon dioxide is exhaled and more oxygen is inhaled for exchange. The oxygenated blood now flows into progressively larger pulmonary veins until four large veins (two from each lung) return the blood to the left side of the heart. The left cardiac ventricle is capable of enormous contractile force and pumps the newly oxygenated blood via the aorta to the rest of the body for distribution to the tissues where the oxygen is utilized for metabolism and carbon dioxide is generated. Thus the cycle is complete and amazingly enough occurs 60 to 100 times per minute for our entire lives.

The diseases that can impair this process are far too numerous to mention and include disorders of the lung, blood elements, cellular dysfunction, and cardiovascular disease. A discourse on those restricted to the lung is stuff of multi-volume texts and is thus not within the scope of this book. Suffice it to say that whatever the lung disease, it must severely affect both lungs for a patient to arrive at the point where supplemental oxygen is required. One can easily survive comfortably on one lung. As I tell my cancer patients:

"God gave you two lungs so that I could remove one for you."

This statement is intended for the patient in whom the removal of a lung is life saving and for whom the lung on the other side is functional. However, the patient with severe lung disease who is dependent on a continuous flow of oxygen-rich air can barely survive an anaesthetic, let alone the removal of one of his or her lungs. Yet to perform the transplant, the first thing we must do is exactly that—remove one of the lungs to make room for the new donor lung. This is the first critical step. Will the remaining lung support the patient until the new lung (or graft) is in place?

During the operation, the patient is supported by a mechanical ventilator. A ventilator is a machine that forces oxygen-enriched air into the lung. Normally we breathe air that has twenty-one percent oxygen capacity, but under mechanical ventilator support we can deliver 100 percent oxygen. Nonetheless, even that might not be sufficient when only one diseased lung is present.

In addition, the heart must now pump its entire output through only half the vessels that were present before the first lung was extracted. In a normal person with healthy lungs, that is not a major achievement because the heart can easily accommodate to twice the resistance. It seems every organ system has a built-in reserve. However, in this situation, because of the pre-existing disease process, the baseline resistance in each lung has already increased considerably. The vessels have been either destroyed or made thickened and less resilient by the disease process. Thus, the strain on the heart may become overwhelming, resulting in a failure to support the blood pressure.

Consider a mechanical water pump. As you increase the resistance of the pipe through which it pumps the water, the chances of the pump's failing and backing down increases. At some point the pump will burn out. As a result, in about twenty-five percent of patients it will be necessary to place the patient on cardio-pulmonary bypass—the so-called heart/lung machine employed for cardiac surgical procedures. And here is a paradox seen throughout medical intervention—a therapy can itself lead to further problems. The bypass machine has its own series of complications, some of which are unique to lung transplantation. So we avoid bypass if possible.

Remember that although medicine can cure disease, everything that a doctor does carries a potential adverse effect. At all times the physician must balance the risk of what he/she does with the potential benefit. A blood transfusion is an example. Such can cause hepatitis or AIDS. It can also be life saving, and thus judgment and timing are required to ensure that patients receive the transfusion when they require it—that is, when the benefit outweighs the risk. Thus the transplant surgeon may try to avoid using cardio-pulmonary bypass in order to not acquire the potential complications it can bring. The attendant problem with this practice is that when bypass is required, it might have to be instituted quickly, a situation that can lead to considerable drama in the operating room—not to mention stress for the surgeon and anaesthetist.

Perhaps an example will illustrate what I mean. Long after the program was established and I was now its head, I recall one young woman upon whom I was performing a double lung transplant. The first lung was inserted without difficulty and all seemed well. During the extraction of the second lung, the anaesthetist informed me that the oxygen levels were falling. This suggested that the new lung was not able to support the patient properly. Such can happen if the donor lung upon which we are now depending for the provision of oxygen has been outside the donor for several hours before we do the actual transplant. As a result of this temporary damage, it might not function sufficiently to maintain adequate oxygen levels as the second of the recipient's lungs is removed. (We usually refer to oxygen levels as the percent saturation of oxygen in the blood stream.) At this point in the operation, I was almost at the point of clamping off the pulmonary artery to her second lung. That manoeuvre often results in an improvement in oxygenation because the entire cardiac output from the right side of the heart would now be diverted to the new lung. So I responded, "I can clamp the artery in a couple of minutes. How bad is the oxygen level?"

"Saturation about eighty-nine percent," the anaesthetist replied from the head of the table.

That is not a critical level, especially in these patients whose bodies are accustomed to lower oxygen levels (less than ninety percent is considered important under normal circumstances). Thus I continued to proceed with the operation, albeit with haste. Within a few heartbeats, I heard:

"Oh shit, Tom, either the saturation is falling rapidly or the monitor lead is displaced [displacement of the monitor on the finger is not infrequent]."

"Okay," I said, "I'll clamp off the artery with my hand." I did not want to take the time to get a clamp around the artery. As I did so, all I could sense from the anaesthetist at the head of the table was frustration and despair.

"The blood pressure is falling fast!" he shouted, followed quickly by, "Heart rate is slowing!"

We were already acting before the second sentence was completed. It was clear that the heart could not take the strain of the entire output going to the new transplanted lung. Clearly the new lung was functioning extremely poorly, likely due to an overly long period of time since it had been extracted from the donor. We had opened the pericardium—the sac in which the heart resides—and were commencing the institution of cardiopulmonary bypass. To do this, we must insert plastic cannulas or tubes into the aorta and heart so that blood can be directed away from the heart to the machine and then returned to the body by a pump after it has received oxygen. This effectively bypasses the heart and lungs and puts them at rest.

Fortunately, before the operation I had asked for a cardiac surgeon to be available should we have difficulties. I called for him now to scrub into the case. The cannula (plastic tube) in the aorta to return oxygenated blood from the machine to the patient went in quickly and smoothly, but the catheter that is inserted directly into the right side of the heart to remove unoxygenated blood to the machine would not pass.

"Oh God," I said, "the atrial cannula will not pass!" As I said this, the cardiac surgeon was coming through the door after a minimal scrub.

I was already doing cardiac massage in between attempts to insert the cannula and was certain that we were in full cardiac arrest as the heart muscle now began to fibrillate.

"Here, I'll do it," my cardiac colleague calmly commented as he pushed my assistant aside. The arriving surgeon always portrays a sense of order and equanimity when he comes to assist a colleague. It's all part of the culture—I would do it, too, when called to extract another from trouble. Perhaps it is part of our attempt to remain cool, knowing that the situation is desperate or we would not have been requested in the first place.

"Damn, you're right; it won't pass for me, either!" he exclaimed. I didn't know whether to be relieved or frightened. It was good to know that it truly was difficult and not just the result of my own inadequacies; but at the same time it was clear that we were losing precious time.

Two more attempts were made with a different technique, both unsuccessful.

"Get me a Pacifico atrial cannula," he yelled. His octaves had risen as he too now sensed the impending disaster. This time it was his as well as my inability to accomplish the lifesaving task before us. After two attempts with the second cannula, he was successful, and cardiopulmonary bypass was started. Oxygenation improved immediately through the machine, and blood pressure was restored. Nonetheless, the patient was supported by a machine, and there was no guarantee that she would be able to manage on her own once we were done.

Emotionally drained, we now had to complete the removal of the right lung and the insertion of the donor lung—potentially two more hours of operating. It was 3:30 a.m. We had been working on this—arranging the case and operating—since 5:00 p.m. the night before. Fatigue was augmented by the disaster we had just narrowly escaped. Luckily, we accomplished the task in another seventy-five minutes and announced that we were ready to attempt to come off bypass. The cardiac surgeon returned to the OR to direct this part of the procedure.

I had never lost a transplant patient in the OR before that night, and prayed silently that this wonderful twenty-three-year-old woman would not be the first one. We had done everything we could, and it was now beyond our abilities to affect the outcome. Gradually, the flow rate on the bypass pump was slowed, while the anaesthetist worked frantically to support the heart and the blood pressure.

Then, "She's in ventricular fibrillation," said the cardiac surgeon. "Paddles up." Just as you witness the electrical shock being applied to patients on medical television shows, so too must we do this in the operating room when the heart fibrillates. After two attempts at defibrillation with the paddles, a normal heart tracing momentarily appeared on the monitor; but fibrillation quickly returned. Full bypass was restored, and all I could do was wait and watch while the anaesthetist juggled various drugs in an effort to produce a response in blood pressure. We tried again to decrease the flow. Ventricular fibrillation followed yet again.

"Paddles up—let's do it again; all clear," announced the cardiac surgeon. His voice was now a monotone. He was in the distancing mode—extracting himself and depersonalizing the experience. The place was becoming very quiet. The scrub nurse whom I had known for fifteen years looked at me with a sympathetic eye over her mask as if to say, "I know how you feel—it's okay. You tried your best."

"There it is!" he cried, "we have sinus rhythm!" The heart was pumping vigorously in a coordinated fashion.

"Thank God!" I said.

"Ditto," was the reply from across the table.

An hour later, I was with the family explaining that although she was stable at present, it would take a couple of days or even more before we would know for sure whether there had been irreparable damage to the brain or kidneys from the insult she had experienced. I went home.

In the morning, her neurological signs were not encouraging, and over the next seventy-two hours they progressively deteriorated. Our elation with the operative success under difficult circumstances was quickly replaced with the full knowledge that she would soon be legally brain dead. What a great family she had! I think they supported me in my anguish more than I did them. With their consent, we finally discontinued life support. I stood at the foot of the bed as her heart slowed and the irregularities in rhythm that characteristically precede cardiac standstill appeared. When it was over, I again reviewed the operative events in order to determine if there had been any indication that we should have intervened sooner with the institution of bypass. I was hopeful that I might find things that the team could do differently the next time, but it was hardly an undertaking to make one feel better. We found nothing, and in the end my cardiac colleague noted, "If you had decided to go on bypass earlier and we had experienced the same technical problems, you'd now be second-guessing yourself for going to bypass too early."

He was right, of course. You are supposed to feel better when time passes, recognizing that there was nothing else you could have done. That rarely happens. You always second-guess yourself. I am doing it now as I think about her for the first time in at least three years. I imagine I always will.

A few more words about the actual operation are appropriate, as it will be important to appreciate these points to fully understand the patient events that follow. Once we remove the recipient's lung(s) the new donor lung(s) is brought to the operating room, having been extracted from the donor and preserved in a cold solution.

The insertion of the donor lung into the recipient involves three important steps. First, the veins draining the oxygenated blood from the lung must be reunited to the left side of the heart. When surgeons unite two ends of a hollow structure, they refer to the final product as an anastomosis. The next step is to reestablish pulmonary arterial continuity so that the unoxygenated blood from the right side of the heart can find its way into the lung. The pulmonary artery, however, is as thin as gossamer and must be sutured with great care. Otherwise, as I have found to my chagrin, the final result looks more like a watering can spout than a conduit for blood. With the completion of these two anastomoses, we are capable of having blood flow through the lung. However, the surgeon cannot permit that to occur without first completing the third and final step—the reestablishment of airflow.

Air arrives in the lung via your windpipe or trachea, which you can feel in your neck. The trachea divides into a left and right main bronchus, one to each lung. The latter continue to divide until the tiny air sacs for the exchange of oxygen and carbon dioxide are achieved. It is, however, the right or left main stem bronchus that must be sutured as the third step (recipient to donor) during the transplant procedure. It is the most technically difficult of the three anastomoses. It is also the portion of the operation that leads to the greatest postoperative problems and in the majority of early cases was the commonest cause of death, including that at Toronto General Hospital in 1977.

The reason for this is that the lung is the only organ in the body to be transplanted without an oxygenated blood supply. All tissues require oxygen to survive and perform their normal functions. We noted earlier that it is in fact un-oxygenated blood that comes to the lung from the rest of the body via the right side of the heart (Figure 1). The blood is oxygenated *in* the lung and returns to the left side of the heart for distribution to the rest of the body. During this distribution of oxygenated blood, the lungs themselves receive oxygen from small arteries (2 to 3 mm in size) that course along the main stem bronchi and hence are called bronchial arteries. These arteries are divided when the lungs are removed from the donor and are too small for re-suturing. As a result, the only oxygen received is from the pulmonary artery itself, which, as we have noted, carries unoxygenated blood. The bronchus is at the very end of this distribution, so that whatever oxygen might have been available would likely have been exhausted by the time blood reaches the bronchial anastomosis. Thus the bronchus is susceptible to a significant injury, as without oxygen the tissue will either die or heal poorly. That fact alone had been the Achilles heel of lung transplantation.

Although the disruption of the bronchial anastomosis (due to poor healing) had been the cause of the majority of post-transplant deaths prior to 1978, there were other points along the course of the transplant procedure and postoperative phase where difficulties had arisen. For example, most of the patients were of necessity maintained on mechanical ventilators for a long period of time following the procedure, due to the fact that the new lungs were slow to recover from the shock of the extraction procedure. There was considerable controversy as to whether this initial dysfunction was the result of poor preservation of the donor lung or early rejection by the recipient. In addition, we speculated, the failure of the bronchus to heal could be just as much a function of the fact that air was being forced into the lungs under pressure from a machine as it was due to the poorly oxygenated blood supply. We mused: could it be both? There was a host of other questions to be answered before another attempt at transplantation was made.

Why was it so difficult to wean patients from the machines? Even when the x-rays were clear and the lungs had apparently recovered, other surgeons had recorded problems in weaning, and thus a prolonged period on the ventilator.

How could one distinguish between rejection and pneumonia in the post-operative period? The x-rays looked the same. They both caused fever and an elevation in the white blood cell counts. What was the best way to approach this problem?

All these things were experienced in that early case of the seventeen-year-old boy that resulted in failure in 1977. Thus, it became clear to the Toronto team that the development of a successful program would not only require some animal experimentation towards a solution to bronchial disruption, but that in addition there would need to be the formation of a strong interdisciplinary team to handle the post-operative phase.

The team members would each be assigned the task of analyzing a particular aspect and problem, so that all facets of the process could come together. Only in this way did it seem that the problems of the past could be overcome in a comprehensive manner. The success of this procedure would require a group of dedicated people—not just one or two individuals. Thus in 1978, Toronto General stopped clinical lung transplantation and retreated to the laboratory and began the arduous process of recruitment and coordination of the team that would finally perform the world's first successful procedure.

CHAPTER 2

The People

In everyone's life there is a time when unique opportunities present themselves. The ambitions and achievements of very different individuals that seemed at one time to be on diverging courses suddenly coalesce. The events that bring everyone together are not always related to the common theme that emerges, and the result may be very different from that intended by the participants. Nonetheless, the product would never have been realized without the efforts of the collective whole. In the summer of 1982, that was really how it was at Toronto General Hospital. Great events and achievements at times were meant to happen. Prior to that time, the ingredients for success were all there—it just needed the spark. There was at that time a collection of individuals at Toronto General whose talents and interest were perfectly matched; they covered the waterfront as far as pulmonary transplantation was concerned.

The "spark" was Joel Cooper, who was both the spirit and the driving force behind the entire project. Driving force is an understatement. Joel walked (or rather ran) in a straight line to his destination and demanded that we all follow. Whether we ran

THOMAS R.J. TODD, MD FRCSC | 19

abreast or behind him, it didn't matter—just as long as we adhered to the logic he pursued. He was frighteningly intelligent and also had the capacity to logically determine the path to the destination he had pre-determined. He could devise a means of solving the immediate blockage in the roadway without losing sight of the goal beyond. He was not a brilliant scientist. He would not discover new knowledge. Rather he was able to take the incomplete information provided by others—albeit at times unrelated to the problem at hand—and reshape and refine it to find what in the end seemed like a logical solution to a vexing problem. He had dogged determination. When the rest of us were ready to quit, he tried harder. He never gave up. If survival at any cost is the banner of the dying patient, Joel Cooper was his standard bearer.

Joel became interested in terminal lung failure during his medical school training at Harvard Medical School and his subsequent residency in thoracic surgery at the Massachusetts General Hospital. While there, he had with several others investigated the possibility of artificially maintaining patients whose lungs had failed beyond their capacity to sustain life. Working with Warren Zapol, he had been involved in the development and clinical application of extracorporeal membrane oxygenation (ECMO). It refers to the circulation of blood outside the body (extracorporeal) into an artificial lung (membrane).

When a patient's lungs fail to the point where they cannot provide sufficient oxygen to support the body's needs (so-called respiratory failure), they are supported by machines called *ventilators* that force oxygen-rich air into the lungs under pressure.

Whereas the air we breathe is composed of twenty-one percent oxygen, the ventilator can supply 100 percent oxygen. For those whose lungs recover or who do not deteriorate further, this is a tremendous advantage, for it permits the physician to keep the patient alive until the lungs have sufficiently recovered to allow the patient to again breathe without support. Basically, it provides the necessary time for therapy to work, or, in some cases, for the normal reparative mechanisms of the body to do their work.

However, there are always patients whose lungs continue to deteriorate to the point where the standard ventilator can no longer provide sufficient oxygen to support the patient. In the absence of an alternative to provide oxygen, the patient would succumb. In 1982, although ECMO could provide such an alternative, it was a controversial intervention and was available in only a few centres worldwide. When Joel first came to Toronto, many greeted his technology with uncertainty. As a young trainee of his, I found this leading edge of critical care medicine the challenge of my life.

The "membrane" of the ECMO is really an artificial lung. Blood is circulated from the patient into a system of silicone tubes that permit the diffusion of oxygen and carbon dioxide across their surface. The system sounds simple but actually involves some complex circuitry (Figure 2). Blood does not "like" to be outside the body. Once removed from the smooth surface of the blood vessel, it clots just as it does when you sustain a cut. If it clots, then the circuit will be obstructed, and flow will be impossible. As a result, anticoagulation of the patient is a necessary evil if ECMO is to be effective. Consequently, spontaneous hemorrhage can occur. Yet this is but one of a myriad of complications that occur because of ECMO. Despite the complications of ECMO therapy, if it is not instituted, the patient will succumb to respiratory failure.

It is a matter of balancing risk versus benefit. A high complication rate seems acceptable when the alternative is death. The difficult part of the process is ensuring that your timing is correct. If you institute the therapy too soon, then a complication that takes the patient's life might have been averted if recovery would have occurred without the treatment. If instituted too late, then the patient could die as a result of your tardiness and

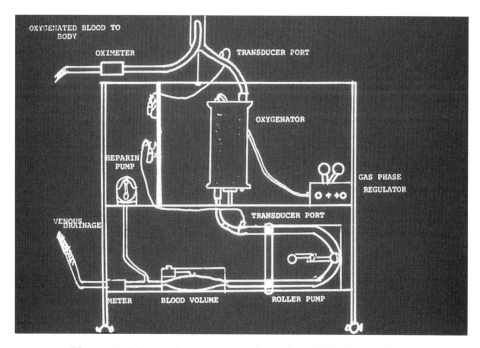

Figure 2. Schematic representation of an ECMO machine.

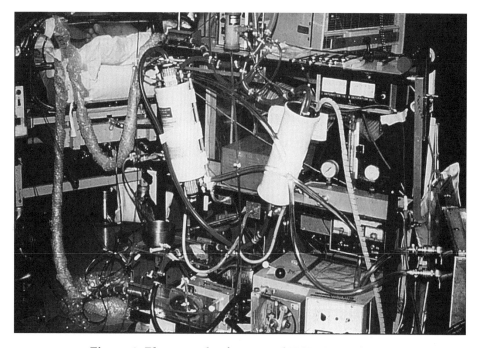

Figure 3. Photograph of an actual ECMO machine.

indecision. This is the problem that critical care physicians and surgeons face daily. Every intervention carries a risk, and one must balance risk versus potential benefit in everything you do.

Joel, in his logical way, and with the assistance of others, circumvented a number of the problems with ECMO. By 1982, we had managed fifteen patients in this manner. Three had survived. Now, that is not a great survival rate, but bear in mind that all of these were doomed to a fatal outcome had the ECMO therapy not been instituted. Joel had also been involved with the General's first attempt at lung transplantation in 1977 described in chapter one. When everyone else was satisfied to accept defeat as inevitable because it had happened to all previous attempts at the procedure, he chose to find the logical solution. He was often noted to quote from Santayana: *"Those who fail to learn the lessons of history are doomed to repeat them."*

He used to drive us residents crazy with that quotation every time we did something that resulted in a poor outcome. However, he lived by his own advice. He recognized that most of the other transplant mortalities had likewise failed because of the difficulty with the healing of the bronchial anastomosis. In addition, he observed, during the autopsy of that unfortunate seventeen-year-old boy in 1977, that the other suture lines or anastomoses between the pulmonary arteries and the veins also demonstrated extremely poor healing. Although they were still intact, the healing was not as good as one might have expected at that point. The bronchial suture line could be explained by the fact that there was no oxygenated blood supply to the bronchus, as we have noted before. But the other suture lines—why should the healing there be impaired? A fair question. While others were shaking their heads in frustration, Joel Cooper was already beginning to seek the answers to the questions posed by the death of that unfortunate patient. All he would need were the people to help him find those answers.

Enter Oriani Lima. Oriani had finished his surgical training in his native Brazil. His interest in lung transplantation was keen;

after hearing Joel speak on the subject, he came to Toronto to pursue his own ideas. He worked with Joel in the Thoracic Laboratories. A gentle and unassuming fellow, he provided a marvelous alter ego to Joel's mercurial thinking. He had great ideas, and Joel had the resources and the imagination to carry them through to fruition. Together they were to conclude that the failure of the generalized healing was actually the result of the therapy in vogue to suppress rejection of the transplanted lung.

At that time, there were two drugs that were utilized in all transplants of any type: Immuran and Cortisone. The latter had been observed by surgeons for generations to impair the healing of wounds. The drug's apparent necessity in preventing rejection had led surgeons to ignore the deleterious effects on healing and to ascribe the poor healing of the bronchial suture line to the absence of an oxygenated blood supply or rejection itself. They simply had not noted that the bronchus was the most obvious area of a generalized poor healing process in these patients. Unfortunately for lung transplant patients, cortisone was also the drug that the majority received to treat their terminal lung disease that had brought them to transplantation in the first place. As a result, patients had been on the medication for months or years before undergoing transplantation.

Dr. Lima performed several autotransplants on dogs—that is, he removed the lung and re-implanted it in the same animal. The importance of that manoeuvre is that rejection is not operative— it is the same tissue just re-implanted as if it were a true transplant. As a result, none of the post-operative problems can be ascribed to the phenomenon of rejection. Lima then treated one group of dogs with the imunosuppressive agents of the day—Immuran and Cortisone—and a second group with cyclosporin, which at the time was the new kid on the block. Cyclosporin, the immunosuppressant that revolutionized the management of rejection, was just undergoing clinical evaluation. The observations in these two groups were startling. The animals that were treated just with cyclosporin demonstrated healing of all their incisions and most particularly healing of the bronchial suture line in a fashion similar to animals that received no immunosuppression at all. The animals treated with cortisone, however, had a marked reduction in the strength of the bronchial suture line. He concluded that cortisone impaired the healing of the bronchial anastomosis (suture line) and thus should be stopped pre-operatively and avoided in the early post-operative period in favour of cyclosporin. We all accepted this as fact. (We would realize eventually that there were flaws in the experimentation; but more of that later.)

Oriani Lima was also concerned that the failure to adequately heal the bronchial suture line might be due to the fact that the lung was, as noted above, the only organ to be transplanted without an oxygenated blood supply. The arteries to the lung carry non-oxygenated blood from the rest of the body. Indeed, blood is pumped through the lungs to become oxygenated. All body tissues require some oxygen to undertake their normal metabolic processes, especially if they become damaged and must undergo a metabolically active process of healing. Thus, if the bronchus were devoid of a rich supply of oxygen then perhaps healing would be problematic. The problem then was how to get oxygen to that bronchial anastomosis. The solution that occurred to Joel and Oriani was the *omentum*.

The omentum is a large apron of fatty tissue in the abdominal cavity that hangs off the stomach and the large intestine. It is rich in blood vessels. It appears like a sheet of fat and blood vessels, with no apparent properties or function (Figure 4). Yet surgeons had been aware for a long time that it appeared to have unique properties, in that when they operated for appendicitis or a perforated ulcer they usually found the omentum had actually migrated to cover the abnormal area. Indeed, it appeared as if it were trying to seal the infected area. More important, it was observed that when you tried to separate the omentum from the ulcer or the appendix, bleeding occurred. That is, the omentum had established a vascular communication

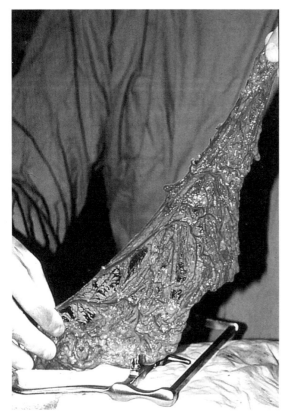

Figure 4. Picture of the omentum, taken during a transplant.

with the damaged tissue. Thus, Joel and Oriani developed the hypothesis that if the omentum could establish a vascular communication with damaged tissue then perhaps it could do so with the bronchus and re-vascularize the anastomosis.

The omentum is flat and large, as shown in the picture, and as a result it can be mobilized and transported with its blood supply intact to other sites. In fact, "tongues" of omentum can be brought up to the neck without too much difficulty. They performed a series of transplants in dogs that conclusively demonstrated that the omentum could re-establish vascular connections with the donor bronchus in a very short period of time. Its use in patients would involve the creation of another incision in the abdominal cavity, but the potential benefit seemed to warrant the extra operative trauma.

Thus, a second important conclusion was reached—not only should cortisone (steroids) be avoided both before and during surgery, but in addition, surgeons should routinely employ the omentum to buttress the bronchial anastomosis. The work of Oriani Lima was integral to the ultimate success of the lung transplant program in Toronto. He would be there to witness the initial excitement. He then returned to Brazil. Unfortunately, the politics and restrictions in his native country would preclude his own participation in such a program for many years.

When it came to the clinical program, there was a stellar array of talented individuals. In 1982, Griff Pearson was the chief of surgery at the Toronto General Hospital and was my senior partner. He was an accomplished thoracic surgeon who had achieved worldwide recognition for his surgical innovation and for the ideas he had spawned for others to build upon. A tremendous motivator, he educated an entire generation of thoracic surgeons who would assume leadership positions throughout North America and beyond. As of this writing, his trainees are in leadership positions at the University of Ottawa, Laval University, McMaster University, University of Pennsylvania, University of North Carolina, New York City, Iowa, Pittsburgh, Japan, Vancouver, Seattle, Harvard, University of Massachussets, Atlanta, Philadelphia, Belgium, and University of Montreal, to name but a few.

Yet it was not his surgical prowess and educational skill that contributed to the events that were to take place. Certainly his technical skills would at times be called upon, but it was instead his sense of altruism and group collaborative practice that provided a concrete example of how the whole process might be orchestrated. Griff had always preached the principle that one should hire a person for the job and then give him his head and let him do things his way; at all times a part of the greater whole of the unit. He never actually said that, but he amply demonstrated it by his everyday actions. He believed that the whole could indeed be greater than the sum of the parts—a difficult philosophy for egocentric surgeons to adopt. He was generous to a fault with his junior members. I remember when he called me to his office to "tell" me that I was to run the new surgical intensive care unit at TGH. He made the appointment and then left the organizational and the operational policies for me to work out. He made Joel the director of the transplant program even though he himself was the senior person and could have claimed the success. He recognized the worth of his partners, encouraged and supported them, and simply expected them to achieve.

During my early years as a member of the group, he called me to the operating room one early afternoon. He was in the midst of a complex surgery upon a Greek air force pilot. The patient had suffered extensive injuries in an air crash several years previously. He had undergone a repair of his trachea as well as reconstruction of his chest wall. Both repairs had been less than perfect despite several subsequent operations. Such cases were referred to Griff from around the globe. There were few surgeons capable of performing the type of surgery that this young man required, and Griff was one. The reason for his call to me that afternoon was that he had an important meeting with the administration in his role as the Chief of Surgery for the hospital. He requested that I take over the procedure, stating that he would return in an hour or so. Delighted to be given this challenging case, I accepted the request enthusiastically.

During the initial two hours of surgery, which was definitely challenging my abilities, I scarcely noted the passage of time. However, by four o'clock in the afternoon, I became anxious for his return so that he might place his stamp of approval on what we had achieved. We were finished just short of five o'clock and I suggested that we page him to determine if we should leave the patient in the room for his perusal. When he didn't answer his page and there was no answer in his office, I broke my scrub and quickly walked down the stairs to the executive suite to search for him. Finding the latter deserted, I returned to the operating room and had the idea that I would leave a message at his home so he might at least be aware of the fact that all had gone well. To my surprise, it was Griff who answered the phone. He was already home. He had simply forgotten about the case after his meeting was concluded. Delighted to find that he had nothing else to do that afternoon, he had actually left early.

Griff is unique. Here he was, operating on a patient sent to him as a last resort from a foreign country. It was a unique and challenging problem, and yet he was content to leave a significant portion of the procedure to his junior partner. Both he and I knew that I would call him when and if the procedure was beyond my capabilities. This attitude permitted all of us to develop our own skills at a pace that could not have been achieved in any other institution at that time. It was this spirit of co-operation and constructive effort that enabled Joel to form a special group of individuals—whose collective strength would indeed be greater than the sum of their individual talents. Griff was awarded the Order of Canada in 2003. He was a true giant in the field of academic surgery.

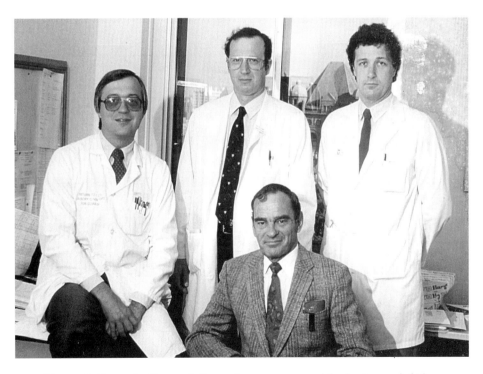

**Figure 5. Toronto General thoracic surgeons, mid-nineteen eighties.
L to R: Tom Todd, Joel Cooper, Alec Patterson,
with Griff Pearson in front.**

Wilfred Demajo, both anaesthetist and internist, is the consummate physician and intensivist—he could do everything but operate. His knowledge base is enormous; he possesses so much information he becomes scary at times. He is Maltese by birth and is affectionately known as "the Falcon." His demeanour matches the label when he is in the intensity of the moment or locked in one of his frequent and emotional clinical discussions or teaching sessions. We arrived at TGH in the same year and month—July 1978—and were both assigned to the intensive care unit. Two Type A personalities with egos a mile long and the desire to prove themselves creates a formula for fireworks. That indeed happened, and for a while we petulantly spent as much energy criticizing each other as we did looking after patients. It was destructive. We owe our friendship and the subsequent development of critical care at TGH to the intervention of one of our colleagues.

One Friday afternoon, he closeted us in the same room and provided the opportunity for us to vent our feelings towards each other. We emerged as colleagues and developed a friendship and professional relationship that created an environment in the ICU that many sought to emulate. We finally realized, as Griff would have told us, that we were far more effective as a team than as individuals. Wilfred was given the task of providing anaesthesia to the transplant recipients. Basically it was his job to ensure that they stayed alive while we did our work. Not a mean task when you consider the fact that the patients were already oxygen dependent and were about to have one lung removed for an hour or so until the new one was sewn in place. He was always there, always keen, and always the one I looked to when the going got tough. I have said that there is only one face I want to see if misfortune should land me in an ICU. That is the Falcon.

In the corridors of TGH, legends are established quickly. One such was Michael Francis Xavier Glynn. Bespectacled, bearded, and appearing as fragile as his patients, Michael was a tower of power, support, and enthusiasm. He was our coagulation expert,

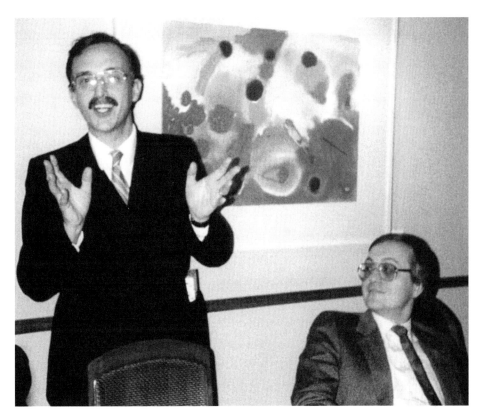

Figure 6. Wilfred Demajo.

and it is really hard to conceive that there will ever be another quite like him. How many times have I stood in an operating theatre attempting to find a mechanical solution to the problem of ongoing hemorrhage that was threatening my patient, only to hear Michael's voice from the door?

"Harrumph . . . Ah, how can I help you?"

My responses were never prosaic or even kindly and usually consisted of something like: "Thank God you are here!" or, "I don't care what the hell you do, Michael, but please do it quickly."

He always did. Clotting is important stuff for a surgeon and Michael took it seriously. It can, however, also be hazardous if it occurs in the wrong place or at the wrong time. We know all about that with the problem of clot development in the leg and subsequently the lungs while flying long distances in our modern world. If clotting occurred in our anastomosis or within the donor lung while it was sitting in a cold bath awaiting implantation, it would be a disaster. Michael's job was to strive for a happy balance. He had to ensure that coagulation did not occur when deleterious, but at the same time had to prevent the patient from bleeding to death.

He did a wonderful job, but over and above all that, he was a true physician. Most hematologists of his expertise will give an opinion in their area but are not personally available on site at all hours of the day and night. Michael was. He was also ready to comment on every aspect of the program and of an individual patient's care, providing new insights and challenging questions. He would arrive in the ICU or operating room with a syringe or IV bag containing something or other to enable us to stop abnormal bleeding. When you asked what this was, he would merely smile knowingly and say, "Just give it— don't ask." I still don't know what I gave on many occasions. It drove nurses crazy and probably would have landed a lot of us in a great deal of trouble if things had not gone smoothly. In fact, it would be inconceivable and unethical today to simply administer a drug without knowing what it was. We trusted Michael, and the trust was well placed. Most of us are replaceable when we pass on from clinical practice. Michael was not—he was truly unique. He died in an intensive care unit at TGH at far too young an age.

Alec Patterson joined the group in 1984. Another student of Cooper and Pearson, and one of my first residents, he provided considerable surgical skill and would eventually take over the program from Joel when the latter departed for the United States in 1988. Alec is one of the finest technical surgeons I have seen. Of the surgeons I have known, he comes closest to the technical wizardry of Pearson. Working in Joel's laboratory with a young surgeon from Edinburgh named John Dark, he perfected the technique of simultaneous double lung transplant. He likewise left Toronto, doing so approximately three years after Cooper to join him in St. Louis. Over the next ten years, many of the innovations in lung transplantation would come from the collaboration of Cooper and Patterson. Together they have established a centre of world renown. Alec has become one the best-known thoracic surgeons in the world.

There were other thoracic surgeons who played a supportive role in the early days. Of these, Bob Ginsberg and Mel Goldberg were the most prominent. They were both based at the Mount Sinai hospital across the street from TGH. They selflessly gave of their time to provide assistance when we needed it most, despite the fact that they gained little recognition outside of our own group. Bob was our initial coordinator when we were still extracting the donor lungs in an adjoining room. He ensured that the timing was correct, cajoling one team to hurry and slowing the other down. A heavy smoker, Bob unfortunately passed away from lung cancer in 2003. He had, however, become one of the world's foremost thoracic oncologists following his relocation to the Memorial-Sloan Kettering Cancer Institute in New York City. Before his untimely death, he was able to witness a spectacular and moving tribute to his surgical career hosted in Toronto and attended by surgeons and oncologists from all over the world. He could not have failed to appreciate the regard in which he was held.

Mel Goldberg had a long-standing interest in transplantation. He had undertaken several laboratory studies to determine the best means of extracting and preserving donor lungs. He and I shared the duties for the donor operation for several years. Mel is one of the most unassuming and pleasant surgeons it has been my pleasure to know. He joined the exodus from Toronto and currently is the head of Thoracic Surgery at the Fox Chase Cancer Clinic in Philadelphia.

One should always save the cream for the last. It seems an appropriate place to discuss them, for they are always the last to be considered in medical drama. They are the unsung heroes—the nurses. Not just any nurses, however, but thoracic and ICU nurses. They are special people indeed. They are different from any of your preconceived notions of a nurse. In fact, their characteristics are so constant that you can pick them out before they even know that thoracic surgery or ICU is their ultimate destination. On several occasions, I have indicated to a nurse from another area of the hospital that he/she should consider working in the ICU because of his/her personality and perceptions. Disclaimers usually follow, but they frequently end up there.

Such nurses are aggressive with their knowledge—a knowledge gained at the bedside from observation. They possess an intuition that is frightening. At the same time, they bring empathy to their practice that wonderfully balances their personalities. Except where physicians are concerned, of course. With us they show no mercy. They like nothing better than to play one-upmanship on the doctor. It is a wise surgeon who

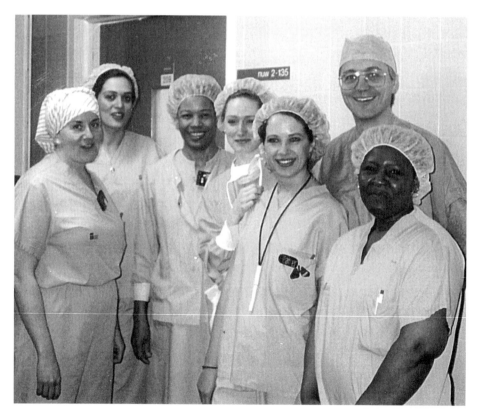

Thoracic Operating Room nurses with the author, 1990.

knows how to give them their just recognition. The residents learn that lesson sometimes late and always hard. Failure to recognize their talent is a prescription for troubled times for that physician. A "me doctor, you nurse" attitude usually results with the doctor in question feeling much less a physician. In the ICU doctors and nurses are in a partnership, and when that occurs, the patients are the beneficiaries.

The nurses in the surgical ICU, the operating room, and the thoracic ward at TGH in those days were some of the best with whom I have practised. When transplantation was thrust upon them, they developed an infrastructure and system of care that was copied across North America. They were our alter egos—cheering us on when our egos were low, cajoling us when we needed it, and criticizing us when we deserved that. One characteristic that they share is that they are nomadic. They rarely stay in one place for longer than three years. Many have gone now, and I remember faces without names and names without faces. I hope that those who have gone are someone else's alter ego now. Such a waste if they are not.

I no doubt miss many here. There were physiotherapists, dietitians, immunologists, and others. They all provided leadership, innovation, and support. One physiotherapist deserves special note. Anne Kuus was and still is as of this writing the physiotherapist assigned to Thoracic Surgery. This diminutive tower of power brings out the hero in every patient she touches, motivating them to do what they consider impossible. I swear she is prescient in her ability to appreciate that something is not quite right in the post-operative course. I often indicated to my residents that when Anne calls and asks for a prompt assessment they would be advised to respond quickly and in depth.

There were many contributors who came later after the first successes and failures. However, in the summer of 1982, all of the above replaceable individuals became irreplaceable as a group; a group that would soon stand the world of pulmonary medicine on its head.

Where did I come in? I sincerely hesitate to discuss myself in these pages, but my children will wonder where I was when all the others were working so hard. Well, I was and am a thoracic surgeon—a student of Griff Pearson and Joel Cooper. Like Joel, I was very interested in intensive care.

One of the defining moments of my career came while still a resident at the Wellesley Hospital in Toronto. I was watching a patient die of respiratory failure in the post-operative period. I can still picture myself sitting on one of the ubiquitous grey metal stools that appear to inhabit every intensive care unit in the world. "Unit" in this case, however, is a bit of a misnomer, as it just consisted of a four-bed area at the end of the recovery room. Surgical intensive care was in its infancy. It was 1972, and surgeons had little or no authority in intensive care, and the ICU physicians of the day had a fatalistic approach to the management of these patients.

That day, I sat on my stool feeling inept, wondering what else I could do for this patient. As I spun the stool repeatedly in half circles I recognized that I did not completely understand the pathophysiology that was unfolding in this unfortunate gentleman. That frustration and the realization of my own ignorance would set the stage for an involvement in critical care over the next twenty-five years. Wilfred Demajo and I later adopted the stance that if you didn't understand why your patient was dying, it was not time to give up but rather to become innovative. That attitude was sorely criticized by several doctors and nurses. They felt that we tried too long and too hard with our doomed patients. They were correct in that we frequently failed to keep the patient alive. But each failure brought new knowledge; each case taught us something more. The patients who benefited from our labours can thank the patients who came before them who showed us the way.

By 1982, I was the director of the new surgical intensive care unit at TGH. Thus my role seemed twofold—to participate in the surgical transplant procedures and to organize and provide a system of post-operative surveillance and support for the recipients. At least that was the idea at the start. However, Joel, my boss, had additional ideas. It became clear after the first transplant success in 1983 that the rate-limiting step in the whole process was donor organ availability.

In those early days, we were bringing all potential donors to TGH for extraction of the lungs. We were concerned that the time from extraction of the donor lung to the time of its implantation in the recipient be kept as short as possible. I thoroughly enjoyed the recipient side of care, and the surgery itself was nothing short of wonderful. Yet I hated looking after donors and wanted nothing to do with the surgery on these unfortunate people. Nothing rational, just emotional hangups that precluded my immediate acceptance of the next role Joel had picked for me.

I was an ICU physician as well as a surgeon and although I dealt daily with matters of life and death, was reluctant to provide ongoing medical care to those whose lives were basically over. They had a heartbeat and other normal bodily functions, but as donors, they were now legally brain dead. They might continue with a functioning body for another hour or another forty-eight hours, but not likely beyond that. But that was just the point. Their functions would start to shut down one after another, and the trick was to keep those organ systems well oiled until recipients could be identified. Donors were and are scarce. Thus, as the attending physician of the donor, one's task was to maintain function with the knowledge that it would cease with organ extraction.

The lungs, we were to learn, are often the first of the organ systems to deteriorate following brain death. In fact, lung function can decrease so quickly after the declaration of brain death, even those functioning supremely well at the time we first heard about them became unacceptable before the donor operation could take place.

Joel requested that the surgical intensive care unit take over the care and direction of the donor lung program. I fought it, putting up the usual roadblocks trying to make it seem impossible. But he knew me too well and steamrolled over my objections to the real problem—myself. So of course the ICU took on the problem. In 1985, it took 14.8 hours from the time of donor arrival in the ICU to the point where the operation could proceed. By 1986, that time had decreased to less than four hours. By then, we were beginning to think of doing the donor operation in the original hospital of the donor; and then the development of novel extraction techniques and means of lung preservation were thrust upon us. But that's another matter and the subject of another chapter.

With all this in mind, I'll return you to 1982. The program team sensed that it was now ready once again to initiate an attempt at lung transplantation. The Surgical Intensive Care Unit had been brought into existence. We waited for the green light and the right patient. Unfortunately, when the light turned green, the right patient was not at the starting gate.

CHAPTER 3

On Our Way

Everyone needs practice before perfection can be claimed. That may seem rather callous and irreverent when applied to people and the treatment of their terminal illness, but the fact remains nonetheless true. As a surgeon, you advance by stages. You spend seven years after medical school learning to be a competent thoracic surgeon before you commence your own practice. The next ten years permit you to develop technical and judgmental skills that you presumed you fully possessed upon the completion of your training. Yet that initial decade of independent practice provides a learning experience that readily dwarfs all the supervised surgical training that preceded it. Experience counts. When you have performed only one unsuccessful transplant, there is still a lot to learn.

By the late spring of 1982, the research in Joel's laboratory under the care of Dr. Lima was beginning to bear fruit. In one of our thoracic group meetings, Joel raised the question as to whether we should now consider reopening a program in human lung transplantation. That consideration led naturally to two problems.

The first was defining the indications for a procedure that had never been successful. From a functional point of view, patients with pulmonary or lung failure fall into two broad categories: those ventilated with a machine and those not.

First, there are those whose inability to exchange oxygen and/or carbon dioxide has deteriorated so badly that they need the support of a mechanical ventilator for survival. Such patients require the insertion of a tube into the trachea either through the mouth or via a tracheotomy that creates a hole in the windpipe through an incision in the neck. That tube is then connected to a machine (ventilator) that supplies oxygen-rich air under pressure. Such patients are almost universally committed to reside in an intensive care unit and often have multiple problems with other organs. There are very few patients provided with such support who can be managed with assistance at home. Patients with Lou Gehrig's disease or spinal cord trauma (Christopher Reeves, the actor, provides a modern celebrity example) fall into this latter group. These latter folks do not have lung failure per se but rather cannot move air into their lungs because of a neurological or muscular disorder. That is, their lungs are perfectly normal but they simply cannot generate the muscle power to breathe. In addition, other organ systems are sufficiently functional as to not demand constant medical attention. Providing them with a "new lung" would not alter their dependency on the ventilator.

However, the vast majority of patients with lung failure are those admitted with acute respiratory failure secondary to some form of lung disease. They are on ventilators for days, weeks, or months as the physicians wait for their disease process to resolve. Unfortunately, the disease that created the problem might be cured but the resultant lung damage could be so severe that the patient does not survive or must be relegated to chronic support with a mechanical breathing machine or ventilator.

As an intensive care physician and a surgeon, I was intrigued with the possibility of transplanting this group of patients. The problem was simply determining when to do so. The point of truly irreversible lung failure was then, and still is, difficult to identify with an acceptable degree of certainty. Indeed, I have witnessed patients maintained on ventilator support for eighteen months with resultant improvement to the point where they became independent once more. In such a case, had we intervened with a transplant, the procedure and its resultant complications would have been, in retrospect, unnecessary. Thus, the question of when to intervene still remains unanswered. When respiratory failure itself is rapidly leading to the demise of the patient despite the use of a mechanical ventilator, it is obvious that a transplant might prove life saving. However, under such circumstances, it would almost certainly be impossible to acquire a suitable donor in time. In addition, many of these patients have experienced the failure of multiple organ systems, which would make the chances of recovery from the transplant even more uncertain. Furthermore, many of these patients have a tracheotomy to facilitate the use of the ventilator.

The establishment of a tracheotomy usually leads to a chronic infection in the airways or within the lungs themselves. In 1982, that seemed to be a tremendous potential problem in a patient who would have his/her immune system suppressed following the transplant procedure. It was generally felt at that time that such patients would quickly succumb to overwhelming infection in the new lungs. For all these reasons, the group of ventilator-dependent patients did not seem ideal.

The second category of eligible patients consisted of those whose lung function had deteriorated to the point where they required constant supplemental oxygen. Although severely limited, they did not require a ventilator. They could be moderately active as long as oxygen was supplied. No doubt many of you have seen such people wheeling their oxygen tanks through supermarkets or along the street. These are the very best of this latter group. The majority of this cohort are sufficiently restricted, even with oxygen, that managing the outdoors, particularly on their own, is impossible. In fact, many physicians would have considered it unethical to institute mechanical support in such patients, because when lung function deteriorates to that point in a patient with incurable chronic lung disease, assisted ventilation will likely be permanent. Thus, as respiratory failure progressed, they would be allowed to succumb to their low oxygen levels, receiving all therapy short of the ventilator itself.

The obvious difficulty with this group was to identify the patient whose life expectancy was so short that transplantation might be a worthwhile option despite the universal failure of the procedure to that point. Yet there are many such individuals who will live in this state for several years, and predicting length of survival is as accurate as weather forecasting. For them, the high risk (at that time a 100 percent risk) became a quality of life decision.

Thus it became clear that both eligible groups presented a dilemma. The first (those with acute lung failure on ventilators) had an extremely poor chance of surviving the procedure, and there was the real possibility that the lungs might have recovered anyway. The second might live for another year or two without the procedure, and thus a failure could decrease their life expectancy. The latter dilemma is not such a problem if the procedure has a high success rate. However, when there has yet to be a survivor, it becomes a hard prospect to sell to the patient and his/her family.

The second problem facing Joel was funding. Because subsequent attempts would be regarded as experimental surgery, there would be no payment for the physicians or for the hospital. As far as the physicians were concerned, funding was of no concern. Remuneration was hardly the reason we had all become involved in this project. Indeed, we were so eager that we might have paid the hospital for the chance to be involved. In 1982, we were quite naïve in assessing the cost to our time and our freedom. The bigger financial concern was the drain on the hospital resource that such an undertaking would create. There were nursing costs, laboratory expenses, drug costs (the immunosuppressive agents were costly); the ICU bed alone in 1982 would cost the hospital in the neighbourhood of $2,500 a day. It was estimated that a single patient would result in an expenditure of $120,000 that could not be recouped from government funding. That all of course presumed that the procedure went well and that the patient did not linger in the ICU for months. Under those circumstances, the costs would be significantly higher.

Such sums do not represent a significant amount of a hospital's budget, at least for one the size of Toronto General. However, the administration was quick to query us as to how many procedures would be required before we had obtained sufficient success that the government might globally fund the undertaking and that third-party payers would not consider it experimental. What success rate would be deemed appropriate—twenty percent? Sixty percent? Twelve transplants would involve approximately $1.5 million in costs to the hospital, presuming that none of them had a prolonged course in the intensive care unit. The latter seemed highly unlikely, given the history of the program.

Several million dollars did seem significant, and we estimated that the pilot project would require close to that number. Beyond that, we were aware of the fact that we had entered times of financial restraint in Canadian health care. Thus there were concerns that even if success did occur, the government would not fund us to a level that would allow the provision of satisfactory care. A government-run health care system rarely welcomes—nor does it encourage—innovation.

Little did we appreciate the extent of financial restraint that was to come, and that such would eventually lead all of us to depart Toronto General. If the proposal to initiate this program had been brought forward for the first time in 1992, it would have gone nowhere. Despite our concern over restraint in 1982, it would seem minor compared with what was to come. It was fortunate for our patients and for Toronto General that we were ready before the days when innovation was considered wasteful.

The summer of 1982 found Joel single-handedly addressing these problems. The rest of us watched and waited and most of the time we simply forgot about the whole thing, immersed as we were in our own practices and issues. It was the subject of occasional discussions, but as time wore on, our interest waxed and waned. Joel was the architect and champion, and had it not been for his relentless efforts, what follows would be fiction. Always ready with free advice, we were convinced that many months or even years would pass before the green light was given.

Joel, however, continued to pursue the gold ring, and as luck would have it, the whole matter of hospital approval was taken out of all our hands. There are, as I have already said, events in our lives that are just meant to happen. When the answers to your difficulties are not found within yourself, they present themselves from without in a seemingly unrelated set of circumstances. Just as the critical mass of appropriate physicians had appeared at the right time, so, too, did the patient and the circumstance. The answer to our dilemma came from Atlanta, Georgia, and his name was Jack.

Jack was a horticulturist from outside Atlanta. He was thirty-one years old. He grew large trees of all sorts, and their care demanded the use of pesticides and herbicides to control disease. Jack frequently employed Paraquat,™ a great herbicide but a potential human poison.

Jack was unaware, as were most of us, that Paraquat could be absorbed through the skin. Paraquat poisoning was generally thought to be secondary to ingestion. Once in the blood stream, it produces damage to major organ systems. First, it causes permanent kidney damage, and second, it generates a severe inflammatory reaction in the lung. Renal failure accompanied by pulmonary failure severe enough to require ventilatory support had been uniformly fatal in patients with Paraquat poisoning. The lung failure was not considered reversible.

That summer, Jack had developed nosebleeds following periods of spraying—a sure sign of Paraquat toxicity. He then presented himself to his local emergency department in Atlanta with a cough, general malaise, and shortness of breath. He was found to have marked impairment in kidney function. His initial chest x-rays demonstrated the patchy abnormalities suggestive of either pneumonia or inflammation in his lungs. He deteriorated rapidly and soon required a mechanical ventilator to support the oxygen levels in his bloodstream. Paraquat levels in his blood were found to be very high. A lung biopsy was performed through a small incision in his chest, and pathological examination confirmed a diagnosis of Paraquat lung disease. His kidneys progressed to complete shutdown and he commenced renal dialysis. In order to remove the Paraquat, the blood was circulated during dialysis through a series of charcoal filters. Although the charcoal absorbs the Paraquat, it is a very slow process. Despite these aggressive and appropriate measures, the physicians in Atlanta were losing ground as far as his oxygenation was concerned. His lungs would soon no longer provide sufficient oxygen despite the use of a ventilator that supplied it in a concentration of 100 percent.

The call to Toronto was made because of our experience with ECMO (extra-corporeal membrane oxygenation), but as well because of Joel's apparent interest in conquering the problems with transplantation of the lungs. In fact, the first call was made to Warren Zapol in Boston, who was at the time the recognized world expert in ECMO. He appropriately sensed that ECMO would provide only temporary support, since the lungs were likely to be permanently damaged. Even if ECMO improved oxygenation, it was clear that a permanent solution would have to be found.

Zapol and Cooper had worked together in Boston, and Warren was aware that we might be ready to again attempt transplantation. Fortuitously, the call was forwarded to Toronto. From the hospital's perspective, all the perceived problems with transplantation became non-existent. As the patient was an American, third-party insurance might cover all the expenses. There were no objections to our proceeding.

Arrangements were made for the air ambulance transfer of Jack to Toronto, and he arrived at 1930 hours on August 24th, 1982. The ICU was literally vibrating with excitement. ECMO was in its own right an unusual therapeutic endeavour, considered the ultimate in physiological support of the ICU patient. Although we had undertaken several ECMO runs over the years, they were sufficiently uncommon and dramatic that this fact alone made for some considerable anticipation. Add to this that the patient was being flown in from the USA and that a lung transplant just might be the end result, and one had ICU nurses suddenly willing to take extra shifts.

A hospital has a grapevine of communication and gossip that challenges radio talk shows. If you have a rumour you wish to spread rapidly through a community, start it in the lobby of a hospital—just pick anyone at random and the "facts" or a slightly altered version thereof will be on the street within minutes. As a result, the halls on the second floor of the TGH and the staff lounges in the unit itself were suddenly occupied with residents and interns who "just happened" to be passing through to see if their patients were developing any problems that their newfound interest in prophylaxis might address. By the time I arrived to undertake the initial assessment and arrangements, it was not difficult to determine the bed assigned to our new patient. One just had to look down the corridor to where the crowd was gathered.

I met with Jack's wife and his family shortly after his arrival. The "quiet" room was filled with euphoria, despite the gravity of the situation. Having been made aware of the dismal if not hopeless prognosis while in hospital in Atlanta, the transfer to Toronto was seen as a panacea. They had assumed success was imminent and were certainly not prepared for the drawn-out saga and the roller coaster of emotion that began that night.

Managing the unrealistic expectations of families is not always easy. You certainly do not want to provide further discouragement and a deepening sense of futility. They must retain sufficient hope such that their distress with the situation does not prevent them from accepting the recommendations you are about to make. At the same time, you want them to be insightful and realistic. The biggest problem for the physician is to recognize that the expectations of the family are vastly different from his/her own; that the family's interpretation of what is said and of what they observe is rarely the same as the doctor's. The more we know, the more we erroneously assume what our patients and their families also know. It leads to an incredible information gap that frequently goes unappreciated by both parties until a crisis develops that brings the misunderstanding to the fore.

I remember a personal experience that illustrates this difficulty. My wife's mother had developed ovarian cancer. After some preliminary and rather debilitating chemotherapy, she underwent surgery to remove whatever residual cancer remained. As the surgery was performed at TGH, I was the first to see her in the post-operative period. After I left the room, I encountered my wife and she immediately asked after her mother.

"She looks terrific," I said with great confidence. "Couldn't be better!"

Indeed, that is how I viewed things from the perspective of a surgeon and critical care physician who daily witnesses patients recovering from trauma greater than what my unfortunate mother-in-law had endured that day. I was being forthright and sincere; very much the factual surgeon.

However, when my wife encountered her mother, her appreciation of the situation was somewhat different. She observed the presence of several intravenous lines, tubes running from her mother's nose and abdomen, various pumps beeping away, and, most important of all, her mother complaining of some significant pain. My wife was not just distressed to view her mother in this condition but also considerably upset with her husband for such a grossly misleading representation of the situation. In fact, when she informed me somewhat later in the day that her mother's condition in no way resembled the situation that I had described, I immediately assumed that complications had ensued. Thus, upon returning to her room later in the day, I, too, was confused to find that she actually looked better than when I had seen her earlier. Our observations and expectations are governed by our preceding experience.

The physicians in Atlanta had prepared Jack's family for his death. However, the family, as is typically the case, assumed that whatever the outcome, it would come quickly. They fully understood the risks; they knew his life was in peril and that the proposed intervention bore little chance of restoring it. However, like most families, they were ill prepared for the not infrequent protracted course of events that unfolds in the management of these complex patients. It is true that some patients with critical illness succumb quickly while others may with reparative surgery rapidly recover in a matter of hours or days to the point where they are no longer in danger. There is, however, an intermediate state wherein the patient lingers amid the throes of a cascade of complications with the outcome continually in the balance. It can go on for a considerable period of time.

Recovery is like the stock market graphs that one sees on the television programs or the prospectus that the financial advisors send you. Progress is rarely a straight line upwards. The line has a characteristic sawtoothed pattern of gains and losses. As with the stock market, before recovery occurs the status of the patient can deteriorate below the levels recorded at the initial presentation. The progress of the patient in the ICU also follows this pattern. This case was certainly to be textbook in that sense.

My initial assessment of Jack Collins revealed that a few adjustments in management could significantly improve his oxygenation. I explained to his family that Jack did not need the

ECMO machines at that point. They were ecstatic. In fact, by morning it appeared that the respiratory failure had reached a plateau. As a medical team, we were grateful for this respite. The entire affair had been initiated very quickly and there were clearly some issues to be determined in the presence of the entire team. There were several members of the team who did not feel that the time was optimal for resuming the transplant program. Others felt that this was not the ideal patient. As he was already ventilator-dependent and in addition had renal failure, the risks of surgery were, they argued, considerably higher.

On the other hand, several of us were of the opinion that the patient was ideal for several unrelated reasons. He had no other alternative; without this procedure, he would succumb. He was young and resilient. Even if we failed, it would be unlikely to create problems for the program, as everyone would expect failure from the outset. One thing, however, was certain. Once we instituted ECMO we were committed to go all the way to transplantation. ECMO was merely a supportive manoeuvre—it would take a transplant to save his life. Thus the news the following morning that ECMO would not be required was met with considerable relief—and not just by Jack's family.

We did institute dialysis to handle his failing kidneys and provided for charcoal hemofiltration to remove the traces of Paraquat still in his system. Certainly transplantation was not a consideration with Paraquat still in his circulation. Its persistence would only ensure damage to the transplanted lung.

Remembering the stock market analogy, however, one will not be surprised to learn that later the same evening I was racing through Toronto streets, ignoring red lights, to get back to the hospital as quickly as possible. Our patient was in trouble, and if ECMO was not established quickly, he would succumb before we had instituted any of the things for which he had been transferred to our hospital.

Because ECMO was a dramatic and unusual intervention with inherent risk, it was always the case that such patients deteriorated to a dangerous level of oxygenation with no further therapeutic options before we initiated therapy. They were always far too precarious to move to the operating room, and so we brought the operating room to them. The ICU is not equipped for surgery in the bed; the lighting is poor, the space inadequate, and the table not conducive to comfort for the surgeon with a bad back. With the patient unstable and threatening to arrest at any moment, and organization less than ideal, pandemonium was usually the order of the day.

Nonetheless, that evening in the ICU we made incisions in the neck and the groin to isolate the jugular vein and femoral artery in their respective locations. Large cannulas were inserted in the jugular vein to drain unoxygenated blood from the patient to the membrane oxygenator. Another large cannula was inserted in the femoral artery to return oxygenated blood to the patient from the membrane. By the time the extracorporeal circulation was established, Jack's oxygen levels were extremely low and his heart had begun to beat erratically. Gradually his oxygen levels rose from those incompatible with life to an acceptable range. With the institution of ECMO we had crossed the "medical Rubicon." A call went out that we urgently required a lung donor—and the lung transplant program was unofficially reopened.

During ECMO, the medical staff were required to be in constant attendance. Thus, we worked eight-hour shifts in addition to our regular days in the operating room and clinics. With five of us familiar with the operation of the machine, we did the extra duty every two days. We waited for a donor, our minds on little else. Joel was like a caged leopard, pacing back and forth between the OR and the ICU.

Because of the risk of infection or bleeding while on ECMO support, the chances of losing a patient increases with time. There were no donors, and every day seemed like an eternity. But on the fifth day a donor was found in Atlanta. The local press there had carried the story of Jack's transfer to Toronto and had noted the need for organ donation. The unfortunate donor had received an accidental gunshot wound to the head. Not only did the patient come from the same city, it became clear that the two families knew each other. There was a poignant moment in the ICU waiting room when Jack's wife received a telegram from the donor's family wishing them success and a future based on their personal tragedy.

In those days we were convinced that the donor lung extraction should take place in our hospital. We were concerned that the time between extraction and completion of the transplant not be longer than two to two and a half hours—the so-called *ischemic time*. Beyond that window of time, there was reason to believe that the donor lungs would deteriorate and not function appropriately. (Laboratory observations in animals had substantiated the concern.) Such a time frame was impossible to achieve if the donor remained in Atlanta. Arrangements were made to fly the patient to Toronto.

If there had been excitement the week before, it now reached a fever pitch. There was a number of legal and ethical issues to consider. The donor was brain dead, but all other organ systems were functional. The removal of the donor organs would lead to the ultimate demise of the patient. If we measure life and death as the absence of the heartbeat, that would only occur in our operating rooms with the extraction of the heart and lungs. It was for this reason that the term "brain death" had been coined. It described a situation wherein the brain was sufficiently damaged that no meaningful recovery could occur.

Every jurisdiction has its own criteria for the declaration of brain death, and as a result we had to confirm that the patient was indeed brain dead after his arrival in Toronto. Our concern for the ethics suggested that those of us doing the transplant and taking care of Jack Collins would have a conflict of interest if we were also the ones assessing the state of the "presumed donor."

A second ICU team was called in to assess brain death and to provide basic support to the donor. The second floor was a buzz of activity and not just from medical folk. The newspapers in Atlanta had been informed of the fact that a donor had been found locally and flown to Toronto. As a result, the Toronto press became aware of the situation, and there was a group of reporters hovering around the emergency room entrance. We even discovered one of them roaming the second-floor corridors dressed as an intern!

Later that night, Griff Pearson and Mel Goldberg performed the donor extraction while Joel and I removed Jack's right lung. I'll never forget the rush of emotion that filled the room when they brought us the donor lung. For me it was the ultimate and defining moment in my career—to be a part of something unique and groundbreaking. For Joel, it must have been well beyond that—he had worked so long and so hard to bring this moment into reality. If the rest of us were excited and proud, for him it must have been several orders of magnitude higher. He deserved this moment and those that were to come.

The lung was gradually sewn into place. We fussed over each missed stitch or avoidable delay, concerned that it would deleteriously affect the result by increasing the ischemic time. The omentum had already been mobilized from the abdomen into the chest, and we carefully wrapped it about the bronchial anastomosis. As the clamps came off the pulmonary artery and blood flow to the transplanted lung resumed, I literally held my breath with anticipation. We had all heard about hyper-acute rejection. The transplanted organ swells and discolours immediately due to the pre-existence of antibodies in the recipient. It is quickly destroyed. I had heard it described. I was not to witness it that night, nor in fact has it been my misfortune to ever see it—although as we will see later, it may have occurred, unrecognized, in another patient. Ten hours after entering the operating room, Jack Collins left it alive.

The next morning I stopped the membrane flow. The new lung was working. I stopped induced paralysis the same day. Paralysis is frequently medically induced in ventilated patients, particularly in severe forms of respiratory failure. It eliminates the patient's own respiratory efforts, reduces oxygen requirements, and, stated simply, makes it easier for the ICU physician to control the ventilation of the patient. Jack began to rouse and move spontaneously. By the next day, we were ready to commence weaning from the ventilator itself. Success seemed around the corner. It was exhilarating and far too easy. I went to a friend's cottage for the weekend. Even though it had been a great thrill, I was happy to be away from it all for a short while.

But the problems came. The first was to be a major surprise. We had daily been monitoring the Paraquat levels in Jack's blood. Indeed, we had already ascertained that they were in the normal range prior to the transplant. Originally, at the time of his arrival in Toronto, we were sending his blood sample to a company in California. This meant that the sample had to be out at the airport by 0630 each morning in order for us to receive an answer the same day. Shortly after his admission, we learned that the same test could be performed in Ontario, a mere one-hour drive from Toronto.

Two days before the transplant was performed, there were no detectable Paraquat levels in the samples sent to both laboratories. The two results were consistent. Yet on September 1st, mere days following the transplant, oxygenation again became problematic and the chest x-ray showed the development of abnormal shadows in the transplanted lung. Several diagnoses were entertained, as the chest x-ray is never wholly diagnostic in and of itself. It merely tells you in pictorial form that a problem exists. Consequently, there was concern that this could be rejection or pneumonia or fluid accumulating in the lungs for other reasons. No one even considered Paraquat—after all, the levels from the Ontario laboratory remained normal. By September 2nd, however, things had greatly deteriorated, and Joel undertook a biopsy of the transplanted right lung. To everyone's surprise, it suggested Paraquat damage. That seemed quite impossible until a sample of blood that had been sent to the laboratory in California as a double check reported high circulating levels of Paraquat. Joel called me at my friend's cottage with the fateful news.

"But that's strictly impossible," I replied. "The levels were normal from California last week before we did the transplant. We removed it all with the charcoal hemofiltration!"

"Well, we've got a biopsy and we have abnormal levels in the blood," he said. "Sounds pretty conclusive."

I sat at the other end of the phone speechless and offering nothing constructive. Joel, as always, however, had a further thought.

"Isn't Paraquat stored in muscle?" he said.

The implications of that insight were staggering. Jack had been artificially paralyzed while on ECMO. In other words, he could not move his muscles. The induced paralysis had been stopped following the transplant and the removal of ECMO support. We theorized that the resumption of muscular activity that occurred once we discontinued the paralyzing medication must have released into the circulation Paraquat that had been stored in muscle. If we were right, the implication was monstrous and seemed dramatically unfair. The entire operation had been foiled by the original precipitating problem. This theory, as it happened, would gain a sound basis after Joel performed a muscle biopsy, the analysis of which demonstrated a large amount of residual Paraquat.

As the situation continued to deteriorate, we had to make a decision as to how far we were willing to go in the management of this unfortunate young man. For the surgeon, this is a frequent ethical dilemma. Your surgery has failed or significant complications have occurred. The chances of meaningful recovery are small, albeit present. When do you stop? When does one make the decision that the patient has been put through enough?

In those days, "stop" was not part of our vocabulary, and in most cases this is still true today. There has been an increasing tendency in the past fifteen years to closely examine such issues and to question the aggressive management of patients whose chances of survival are indeed low. The ethical dilemma is how to measure the chance. The situation is further complicated by the fact that all patients are different and the expectations and concerns of their families are vastly different. One must remember that in the ICU situation, it is the next of kin who provides the surgeon with consent to carry on with procedures and to initiate new treatments. The patient is unconscious or so significantly sedated that he or she is not legally able to make the decision, even if he or she appears to understand the discussion. In this era of advanced life support, it is not uncommon for the relatives and the physicians to be in disagreement as to whether treatment should be continued or indeed what treatment should be given. It is common for members of the medical and nursing professions to be at odds with each other over the continuance or discontinuance of therapy.

Adequate communication is the key to resolving these disagreements. In my own experience, a detailed and patient explanation of the pros and cons accompanied by the setting of goals usually ensures that the medical team and the family are functioning as a single unit. In fact, the interaction that is usually more difficult to resolve is the disagreement between members of the medical team.

As a result, Joel was naturally encountering a variety of opinions.

There followed another long conversation between the two of us—hospital to friend's cottage. It was apparent to Joel that ECMO would soon be required once again in order to maintain sufficient amounts of circulating oxygen. But it made little sense to reinstitute this therapy if there were no long-term solution. Accepting defeat was difficult. He was hesitant (a very unusual circumstance for the usually loquacious Cooper); and then haltingly said: "This may sound crazy, but we could always transplant the other lung."

What sweet music that was to my ears. "Joel," I exclaimed, "that's fantastic. Of course, why not? We've come this far. We might as well go for broke."

It was clear that Joel had already decided to proceed not only with ECMO once again, but to also look for another donor and transplant the left lung. It was nice, however, to have your opinion sought. That day I learned a lot about decision-making, but also something about leadership.

ECMO was re-established on September 3rd. All the Paraquat was eventually removed through the charcoal filter, and again we waited for a donor. Once again we returned to our frequent eight-hour shifts supervising the machine, and the days dragged on. However, the press in Atlanta became active. Six days into the ECMO run another donor was flown to Toronto from Atlanta. He was a victim of lead poisoning apparently acquired from the ingestion of homemade alcohol. Although his lung function appeared optimal in Atlanta, it became evident upon arrival in Toronto that significant deterioration in his lung function had occurred during the transport. His blood pressure had fluctuated widely during the trip—not an unusual circumstance when brain death has occurred. The problem was that he had been given a significant amount of intravenous fluid to support the blood pressure. The lungs had filled with fluid, and despite our efforts to improve the situation, pneumonia supervened. It became clear that this donor would not be suitable. He was flown back to Atlanta for burial. The disappointment for all was tremendous and appeared to the team to be the ultimate rejection of our efforts. But we were short on experience in the transplant game. As we were to learn, such disappointments would become commonplace.

The wait resumed. As if we needed more to contend with, the press in Toronto and Atlanta constantly sought information on our now famous patient. We were hounded over the telephone and in front of the hospital. Articles appeared in the local Toronto papers and there was intense interest amongst

Torontonians themselves. We received several calls about donors. But none were satisfactory.

One night while watching the late-night news with my wife, I received a call from the answering service of the hospital. They reported that there was a frantic man on the telephone waiting to speak with me. When I asked who the individual might be they simply answered that he was greatly distraught about the transplant problem at the Toronto General. Would I please take the call, as he had continued to ring them despite their efforts to put him off? She patched him through to my home. The poor fellow was standing in a telephone booth on Spadina Avenue ready to offer one of his lungs for the sake of our patient. He was so emotionally caught up in the drama unfolding at the hospital that it was only with considerable persuasion that I was able to convince him that such was not only illegal but also unlikely to work, as Jack had a rare blood type. The latter was not quite true, but it did get me back to the National News with some assurance that the caller's concerns had been laid to rest.

There followed a further twelve days of waiting after the Atlanta donor had been found to be unsuitable. On the nineteenth day of ECMO, Atlanta called with their third donor. Given the problems experienced with the transport of the last donor, we decided that one of us should fly there and assess the donor on site. If satisfactory, we would then be able to personally supervise the transport and ensure that donor maintenance was undertaken exactly according to our own set of guidelines. As a result, that afternoon I boarded a Lear jet with a respiratory technologist. I did not know it then, but this would be the first of many flights I would make as the program expanded and my role with donors increased.

The unfortunate donor was brought to a small airport on the outskirts of Atlanta. Today I have not the slightest idea of the name or location of the airport. All I remember is that it looked terribly small from the air, and the pilots were joking about the fact that they were unsure if jets actually landed there. I also recall reaffirming my distaste for flying as we plunged out of the sky at an incline. The Lear came to a stop not far from a large Winnebago-type vehicle parked on the Tarmac. Whoever was in charge was obviously *not* in charge, as there was a crush of reporters and sightseers around the vehicle. I was besieged with cameras and questions. It did, however, serve to heighten the excitement and enjoyment of the moment.

Ushered inside, I was astounded to see what was referred to by the team accompanying the donor as their "trauma bus." Canada had—and has—nothing like this. It was a fully equipped emergency room, complete with medical gases, suction machines, operating table, and ventilator. The walls were stocked with enough supplies to handle the casualties of a major conflict. I felt that it would do nicely in replacing my outdated operating room at Toronto General! As I began to envy the resources of the Americans, I had to remind myself that it is the people, not the place, that make the difference. I would come to say that frequently over the next twenty years, always ignoring the obvious rebuttal that the people *and* the place together might be the best of all.

The donor/patient had sustained a spontaneous cerebral hemorrhage and had been declared brain dead by two neurologists at the hospital in Atlanta. All the x-rays and reports had been made available to me, and there was a nurse and a paramedic ready to inform me of his condition. They were busy continuously recording the vital signs.

After assuring myself that the patient was indeed stable, I turned my attention to his chart and read through the saga of his emergency room admission and the eventual declaration of brain death. But I was most concerned with the size and function of his lungs. A review of the x-rays really couldn't wait, and I read the chart as quickly as I could. The trauma bus was certainly well equipped but there was no x-ray viewing box. I had to hold the films up to the light of the window to properly assess the lungs for abnormalities and to measure their size. The initial attempt to do so was rewarded with the flash of several cameras.

I returned to review the chart while someone in apparent authority went off to clear the crowd from around this leviathan vehicle. When finally able, I was reassured on review of the films that the lungs "looked" perfect and that the size would be no problem for our waiting recipient. The blood gas analysis also verified that lung function was excellent. The settings on the ventilator verified that the lungs were compliant to the volume applied, suggesting that there was no sign of difficulty moving air into the lungs. Finally, I turned to the patient himself, and mindful of the problems with the last donor and the expectations that had been placed on me to deliver this one in exemplary fashion, took the time to be thorough.

Last of all, I undertook a bronchoscopic examination of the airway. That involves inserting a fiber-optic light source down the tube in his trachea. Such permits one to examine the condition of the airways themselves, to record whether the secretions appear infected, and also to sample the latter for culture. We had asked for the bronchoscope to be present ahead of time. The way it was handed up to me suggested that this, too, was an integral part of this mobile operating theatre. Again I felt like the country boy amongst the wealthy cousins. We always performed a bronchoscopy to be sure there was no specific abnormality that might preclude the transplant, such as severe bronchitis and infected secretions. In addition, we frequently discovered surprises such as aspirated teeth and other foreign material. On this occasion, all was well, and I felt certain this was indeed the ideal donor for Jack Collins.

With my examination completed, we arranged to move the patient to the waiting Lear. The time outside an ICU provides a real challenge for the physician and paramedic. Indeed, the trauma bus sitting on the Tarmac of the Atlanta airport was the equivalent of an ICU. But outside in the sunshine, or even on the plane, you no longer have the sophisticated alarms and monitoring equipment reporting the vital signs and alerting you to significant changes that require your immediate attention.

In the twenty years since this event took place, those portable systems have improved dramatically; but in 1982, they were less than ideal. Support systems and specialized equipment were minimal. In the Lear, I had all the drugs that we "thought" we might need, an ECG monitor, and a defibrillator, but little else. I prayed that I would not have to use the defibrillator.

A Lear Jet is not spacious. To those of us from lower/middle class backgrounds, the term "Lear Jet" implies opulence and engenders visions of luxury and space for air travel. It's not—it's just a small plane with a few seats. It is so sleek and trim that you can't stand up inside. We normally removed all but two seats during patient transfers in order to accommodate the stretcher. Once the stretcher is in place, the only means you have to move from one end of the aircraft to the other is by crawling over the sides of the stretcher, hoping that you do not entangle yourself in the intravenous tubing.

I had run a cardiac arrest while aloft in a Lear during an ICU transport and did not relish a repeat performance. Spare oxygen tanks and intravenous bags as well as drugs were stored behind our seats in the rear of the plane. In this fashion, the respiratory technologist and I would attempt to keep all systems functioning—not just satisfactorily but perfectly. I was very aware of the fact that this was not a short trip and that we would have no access to laboratory results en route.

Despite all my concerns, we arrived back at Toronto General in apparent good shape, at least as far as I could appreciate from the systems I had to work with. Upon arrival at Pearson airport, I telephoned the hospital that we were on our way. As a result, most of the Thoracic Division and a goodly number of the ICU staff greeted me when we got off the elevator on the second floor. I was elated to arrive safely and with great pleasure announced that I had provided them with the perfect donor, and further suggested that we should transport donors in this fashion from now onwards. In retrospect, I can now appreciate the old adage that you should be careful what you wish for, because you just might acquire such. The truth of this will become apparent later.

A welcome cup of coffee in the ICU lounge followed, during which I related with relish all the above happenings to the nursing staff and physicians who had gathered there to hear the tale. The attention was most gratifying. The anaesthetist to whom I handed over care of the donor poked his head in the door, poured himself a cup, and with a malicious grin that my egocentric stupor overlooked, said, "How's the coffee? Must seem pretty good after that long trip."

"Great!" I replied, oblivious to his tone.

"That's a great donor you brought us, everything looks terrific—blood gases are fantastic and he's stable as a rock."

"Thanks, John," I said, and then foolishly quipped, "But you know, sometimes it takes the 'A' team to make sure things come out all right."

"Yeah, I guess you're right," he replied. "He's perfect. The only problem is, he isn't brain dead."

My mouthful of coffee erupted out of my nose and down my surgical scrubs. This was more than a little embarrassing. I had flown to Atlanta and brought back a brain-dead donor who wasn't brain dead. I had taken everything into consideration. Everything. However, I had presumed that the Atlanta physicians had applied all the proper criteria for the declaration of brain death. As a result, in my examination of the patient, I had not done a full neurological examination. That had seemed rather unimportant in terms of supplying a good set of lungs.

"What do you mean he's not brain dead? That can't be," I said, hoping that somehow I could prove John wrong.

"Well," John replied, "how is the fact that he moved his hand up to his face to ward me off when I was removing the tape around his endotracheal tube?"

John had just described purposeful movement. My embarrassment was complete. There really didn't need to be any other test to unsettle everything. Purposeful movement was an indication of persistent cerebral function. My humiliation was magnified when we had to cancel the operating room, send home the OR nursing staff and inform the recipient's family that things had been "postponed."

My discomfort, however, was nothing compared to that experienced by the physicians in Atlanta who were given the task of explaining to the family of the donor the reason why the return of their loved one for burial would be delayed a while. To this day I have no knowledge as to what they said or even if they were forthright in their explanations. Fortunately for me and them, "delay" was the correct term.

Although the donor was not legally brain dead at the time of his arrival in Toronto, the extent of cerebral injury was deemed by our neurologists to be unrecoverable. They felt that it would be only a short time before our criteria for brain death were satisfied. We waited through the night, hoping that the lungs would not deteriorate in the interval. By morning the man from Atlanta was indeed brain dead by Canadian standards. Lung function had been preserved throughout the night and we proceeded with the transplant and considerable face saving for me.

The transplant of Jack's left lung proceeded uneventfully and his post-operative recovery was as encouragingly rapid as that following the first transplant the month before. Membrane oxygenation was discontinued. By October 6th, we commenced the task of weaning him from the mechanical ventilator.

There are several ways of accomplishing this, and every ICU and individual intensivist has his or her bias as to what works the best. Basically, however, one allows the patient to do progressively more of the work of breathing by incrementally decreasing that of the ventilator. If our progress since the second transplant had been rapid, the wean from the ventilator was painfully slow. Oxygenation was superb, but when removed from the ventilator and asked to breathe on his own, Jack seemed incapable of generating sufficient force to move adequate amounts of air into his lungs.

We were not, however, deterred or discouraged, as this phenomenon is quite common after a prolonged illness because of attendant muscle weakness that accompanies such a devastating and prolonged hospitalization. Jack had been critically ill for a long time. It was now October, his chest x-ray was clear, and we all felt that it was just a matter of time. There was a short bout of pneumonia, but everything else indicated that all was well, especially when we remembered where we had been earlier in the fall. We explained to his family that we all had to be patient. The stock market analogy was repeated frequently. By November 2nd, he managed to breathe all on his own for forty-eight hours.

But he failed again. I was struck by the fact that the coordination of his respiratory muscles was unusual but merely assumed that this reflected misuse and fatigue. I had observed that before. We had expended so much time and effort in navigating new territory, that during this period of his convalescence we lulled ourselves into thinking that he was at this point just another patient recovering from respiratory failure. Our brains were in vacation mode for a while, as if they were tired of pushing their perceptions beyond the here and now. The thought that there was something novel operating in this case simply did not occur to us.

Vacations do eventually end. Finally, we began to question if there was something else amiss. Were we missing something? The search began in earnest. Bronchoscopy verified that the bronchial suture lines were both healing without complication. We could find no evidence of infection. All the tests we could perform on the lungs themselves continued to come up normal, despite multiple repeats of the same analysis. All this once again led to the conclusion that after all he was just weak. But why for so long?

It was Michael Glynn who made the observation. We found him examining Jack one morning while we were making rounds in the unit. He caught up to me in the hall.

"Tell me, Tom, the muscle wasting that comes with nutritional deficiency, doesn't it affect primarily large muscle groups?" he queried, knowing the answer himself.

"Yes, that's true, Michael," I said.

"Have you noticed Collins' hands? The small muscles are extremely wasted."

He was right as always. On further examination, we verified his observation. There was considerable decrease in the bulk of the muscles of his hands, something that is not usually seen in patients who are critically ill and nutritionally deficient on that basis. Although we had been supplying Jack with supplemental nutrition from the first day of his arrival in our hospital, we would still expect considerable weight loss during a prolonged and complicated course such as his. But one does not see wasting of the small, so-called "intrinsic" muscles of the hand. The entire clinical picture now began to make sense. It was his muscles, after all. He simply couldn't exert enough strength to breathe!

Tests of neuromuscular function followed, and a muscle biopsy was finally done on November 17th. The latter demonstrated that muscle fibres had been destroyed and replaced by fibrous tissue. We presumed that this was the result of the Paraquat. We had learned to our dismay after the first transplant that Paraquat was concentrated in muscle. However, to our knowledge no one had ever recorded that it could produce irreversible muscular destruction. It seemed reasonable to presume that no one had lived sufficiently long for it to come to light. In the past, if the patient did not die of renal failure, then the lung destruction would be fatal. Hence there would be no opportunity to witness the deterioration in muscle function.

On November the 19th, the realization that Paraquat had won was devastating. We had gained anatomic and physiological success, but our patient would never be free of the ventilator unless the biopsy was wrong and there could be some recovery of muscle. With his muscles destroyed, Jack would always be incapable of breathing on his own. He was committed to the support of a mechanical ventilator.

As I have noted before, there are patients who live for long periods of time with the assistance of ventilators. In fact, at

Toronto General we had looked after a wonderful woman who had lived in our intensive care unit for over twenty years inexorably tied to her machine. Nonetheless, she had for a period of time worked as a transcription clerk for medical records. She had her own room adjacent to the ICU, complete with refrigerator and her own television. I recall one year her attendance at the ICU Christmas party at Casa Loma, an old castle in the heart of Toronto. I vividly remember watching her at the dinner table as the waiter approached to serve wine. Certainly he might have been aware that there was something unique about this table by the presence of the small green machine behind her chair, but he was definitely unprepared for the sudden appearance of a small catheter in the hands of this coiffed and well dressed lady as she threw back her head and rammed it down her tracheostomy amid the sound of mucous being suctioned from her airway. The whole scene was intensely surrealistic.

But patients like Bernie (short for Bernice) are rare. There was little prospect that Jack Collins could achieve anything approaching this quality of life, let alone any expectation of longevity. His immunosuppression in the face of a chronic tracheostomy would, we felt, predispose him to recurrent lung infection and eventual death from pneumonia. The news was a major disappointment to the team that had worked so hard over 2 ½ months. We had all lost patients before and had shared the pain of grief with their families—but this went beyond that. It was like running well out in front of a horse race only to stumble just before the finish line with your favourite horse lame and about to be destroyed. Except in this case, it is a man who has come up lame with no options, a man whom you have come to know as a person; and, more important, who has become a symbol of your greatest ambitions.

The family was let down by notches. No one had the will to lay it on the line all at once. It seemed too harsh, and in retrospect I think we always hoped that perhaps we were wrong.

We had snatched him back from death so many times—maybe there was another life in him yet. Joel called other North American centres searching for information on Paraquat and its effect on muscle. There did not appear to be anyone who could provide advice and information, and certainly no one with any experience to comment on prognosis. For some time, I was convinced that any day we would come up with some other innovation—yet another idea. He was still alive and with excellent lungs, and I reasoned that time would provide answers and solutions.

But no solution was to come. There was a time as the next week progressed that chronic ventilator support in Atlanta was considered. It would certainly be easier for the family to have him at home. That, too, was to be denied.

On November 25th, there was a sudden collection of a large amount of blood in the tracheotomy tubing. Joel happened to be in the unit at the time and quickly recognized that a communication had developed between the trachea and a major artery (the innominate artery). This is a recognized but unusual complication of a tracheotomy and prolonged ventilation. The appropriate life-saving measures were undertaken, and Jack was rushed to the operating room, where Joel sutured the offending artery. This operation involves in part the actual ligation of the innominate artery. Unfortunately, this artery gives rise to the right carotid artery, which supplies blood to a large portion of the right side of the brain.

We were familiar with this complication. In fact, Joel had written a paper on the subject that detailed the principles of successful treatment. The paper was noteworthy in that we had never lost a patient to this complication, and none of our patients had sustained neurological damage from the ligation of the artery. There are other arteries supplying the brain that in all our previous experience were obviously equal to the task of maintaining adequate blood flow to the brain after the innominate artery was ligated. The vascular connections within the brain between the various arteries are extensive, and if the patient is young and without arterial disease, these interconnections can maintain a sufficient blood supply to remote areas even when one of the major vessels is occluded.

That day, this was not to be the case and again, and for the last time, fate seemed destined to condemn him. Although the operation went smoothly and the hemorrhage was contained, he did suffer extensive brain damage. By November 28th, two electroencephalograms failed to show any signs of electrical activity in the brain, and it was determined that, like the two donors who had provided him with lungs, he, too, was brain dead. Unlike them, he did not serve as an organ donor. It seemed like enough had happened. It was time to just close the book.

In some ways it was almost a relief. Since the diagnosis of Paraquat muscle damage, our daily visits to Jack's bedside had been increasingly difficult. Nothing is more frustrating for a surgeon than to continue a charade of hope when in his heart he realizes that there are no further therapeutic options, that the bag of tricks is empty at last. Nonetheless, following his death, a pall that was palpable fell upon the surgical ICU. From orderlies to nurses to surgeons, the depression was something I had not seen before, and have not seen since, in my years of working in the ICU. The despondency was enormous, and for several days there was a general reluctance to discuss the matter in any detail. Perhaps we all felt that we had lost something of ourselves—of our own hopes and dreams—in the passing of that one man. I have certainly witnessed episodes of greater emotional lability, greater demonstrations of grief and anger. But this was exhaustion and a very real sense of futility. We felt cheated and beaten. It was personal.

As is so often the case, the passage of time provided relief, and life returned to normal both in the Unit and within our thoracic practice. As discussion of the case was undertaken in an objective fashion, the positive side emerged. We had actually transplanted lungs and avoided the dreaded complication of bronchial anastomotic disruption. We had experienced no operative problems. The post-operative care and the education it had provided for us all was unique.

The family had consented to an autopsy. It revealed several important things. First, overall healing was excellent, confirming, we felt at the time, the observations of Oriani Lima that the avoidance of steroids in the first three weeks was important. Second, the right bronchial suture line had actually partially separated. Despite this, the integrity of the airway was not lost— the omentum had contained the dehiscence and prevented extension and perforation, the expected sequelae of such a complication. Thus the autopsy convinced us that had it not been for the Paraquat itself, success would have been realized.

We were about to learn, however, that it was not quite that simple.

CHAPTER 4

Cameron and Linda

The first time I saw Cameron Evans was on ward G South—the respiratory medical ward at Toronto General. The ward no longer exists. It was in the old College Wing, the original building when the hospital first opened over a hundred years ago. The restrictions of government funding and the "down-scaling" of the 1980s and 1990s led to a reduction in beds of almost fifty percent at the General. It was only natural that the oldest parts of the hospital would be the first to be closed to patients. The last time I was there it had, not surprisingly, been converted to an administrative area. There have been so many administrative areas created out of former wards that one wonders how we managed to provide adequate patient care before the administration became as bulky as it is today.

As stated, it was the oldest part of the hospital, with narrow corridors, high ceilings, and small, ineffectual lights that cast long shadows at the end of the day. Its physical appearance very much suggested the images of the old-style hospital in that there was a sunroom for patients at the end of each corridor, private rooms at one end and large four-to-five-bed rooms at the other, the two areas separated by the tiny nursing station.

Although to the casual observer it appeared past its prime and mired in another age, to those of us familiar with its history there was a constant sense that events of import had occurred in these very halls and alcoves. Banting had roamed these hallways. Many greats of Canadian surgery had commenced their careers trudging up and down the same steps that carried me forward to my first meeting with Cameron. In fact, the stairways are scalloped in the centre and worn to a sheen on the edges. I liked the place. It made me feel that I was part of a continuum when I was there, that there was a richness of medical history and personal events that lay hidden in time, untold.

Nonetheless, as you walked onto the ward, you passed small room after small room housing patients in various stages of breathlessness, with oxygen masks or nasal oxygen tubes. You could not avoid the patient stares for, unlike the rooms of today, they all had windows that faced out onto the corridor. The nursing station was extremely small and bore no resemblance to the large complexes of today. It comprised a counter about ten to twelve feet long with some chairs and a chart rack behind it. But then this ward was constructed in the days when nurses actually spent some time in the rooms with their patients rather than sitting glumly and unresponsively at a desk writing interminable notes. That's where I was that day I first met Cameron; I was leaning on the counter, telephone at my ear, answering the one hundred and tenth page of the day.

Cameron was jauntily strolling down the hall pulling his oxygen tank behind him. Pulling an oxygen tank in such a fashion is no mean task, but Cameron did everything with gusto. He had a smile as big as his face as he teased one of the nurses and waved at the window of a fellow patient. He was tall, very thin, with a long face, and was all of nineteen years old. I could see the nurses speak to him and point at me. His smile left him for only a moment and then it quickly returned. He heightened his pace towards the desk.

"So you're Doctor Todd!" he blurted out enthusiastically. "I've been anxious to meet you."

I was indeed three days late. Cameron had known for some time that his doctors were considering him for a lung transplant. I was the first member of the team to arrive for an interview. I realize now that three days must have seemed like a long time to wait for such an interview, whereas for me it was another task to try to fit into a twelve-to-sixteen-hour day. In those days, we all saw the potential transplant candidates separately and then individually provided an assessment of suitability to Joel.

Cameron had a disorder called primary pulmonary hypertension. It is idiopathic. The latter is a medical term applied to a condition when we don't know the cause. (I have often wondered if the first four letters of the word imply more than ignorance as they form the bulk of another rather unkind word associated with an individual's lack of knowledge.) In this condition, the walls of the pulmonary artery become progressively thickened and obstructed. As a result, oxygen is faced with a thicker membrane to traverse as it struggles to diffuse from the terminal airways to the red blood cells within the artery. The pressure in the artery continues to rise as the thickening and obstruction increase until finally the right side of the heart fails, as it can no longer pump blood effectively against the resistance. Under such circumstances, there are times when the right ventricle fails abruptly. The patient may faint. Such "grey-outs," as they are called, usually signal the terminal stages of the disease. Cameron had experienced this on three occasions and he knew what the symptom portended.

His handshake was just as strong as his smile. I thought that he was euphoric as a compensation for the emotional strain that he must have felt. I was pleased to subsequently learn that my initial impression was wrong. This was not euphoria—it was simply Cameron, the bravest nineteen-year-old I had ever met. This was a young man who as he approached death had taken a major bite out of life. I was to talk to him on many occasions. His desire for specifics of medical information was inexhaustible. He knew that Jack had died the previous fall and was very much aware of the fact that lung transplantation had yet to be successful. Yet he was eager to proceed.

Unfortunately, Cameron's case was presented to us shortly after our Paraquat patient had succumbed. Joel was again in the midst of negotiations with our hospital administration. We were somewhat gun-shy and concerned that Cameron might not be the ideal candidate that could make our program a success. His heart was definitely impaired. Would it function normally again once the diseased lungs were removed and the high pressure was alleviated?

To further complicate matters, it was at this time that heart/lung transplantation was enjoying the centre stage of medical progress. The surgical team at Stanford had pioneered the technique in their animal laboratory and had performed several transplants of the heart and lungs together in man with astonishing success. In fact, the operation was thought by many to represent the final nail in the coffin of isolated lung transplantation.

There was good cause for that impression. Not only was it a proven success, but it also offered a means of monitoring rejection that was not available to lung transplants undertaken without the heart. Because the heart is also transplanted, a catheter could be inserted into the jugular vein in the neck and under x-ray guidance advanced into the cardiac chambers. Through the catheter one can pass a small forceps and obtain a small biopsy of the heart muscle. Tissues that are rejecting have a characteristic appearance under the microscope. With this technique, cardiac biopsies could be performed as often as necessary, providing a ready means of determining if rejection is imminent. This was not possible when the lungs were transplanted by themselves.

That this means of obtaining a biopsy would not necessarily assist in the diagnosis of lung rejection was not appreciated at that time. We simply assumed that if the heart and lungs came from the same donor, then the two organs would reject simultaneously. We did not know then that the heart could be normal while the lungs were rejecting. However, we did know that if you transplanted the heart and both lungs to a patient who only really needed one new lung, you were preventing the use of the other lung and the heart for two other possible individuals awaiting a transplant.

Consequently, the major disadvantage of heart-lung transplantation was the fact that a patient with lung failure and a normal heart would have his native normal heart replaced by that of the donor. Today it seems ludicrous that one would consider removing a patient's normal heart only to replace it with that of a donor. However, the procedure had been designed in this fashion for two reasons.

First, as noted above, the heart would not infrequently be failing at the time of transplantation, due to the high perfusion pressures through the abnormal lung. We had yet to learn, although several of us suspected, that the heart was capable of complete recovery once the high resistance from the diseased lung was removed. Second, the technical difficulty of heart-lung transplantation was far less than that of performing a single lung transplant. To fully understand the latter statement, consider a car engine. Although replacing the entire engine is a radical step, it is not as technically challenging as replacing a small, hard-to-get-at part. To replace that part, you will require specific expertise and equipment. There is more finesse and technical dexterity required than in replacing the engine if you are to avoid damage to other parts of the engine. However, would you even consider replacing your engine when all you need is a new starter motor or water pump?

Thus, as the weeks of Cameron's evaluation dragged on, the lung transplant program was itself undergoing rigorous analysis. As one of our residents asked me one day on rounds, "Why are you persisting with an operation that has never and likely will never work, when there is a viable alternative? How can you ethically offer this operation to Cameron? He has at least a chance if you send him for a heart/lung transplant."

Our supportive arguments appeared more and more theoretical. That was certainly the substance of my many conversations with Cameron. He was on the brink and deserved every scrap of information available. Consequently, in March we decided to refer him to Pittsburgh for consideration of heart/lung transplantation. Pittsburgh had recently started a heart/lung program, and, although not as successful as Stanford, it was clear that they would take him on at an earlier stage. The waiting list at Stanford was long, with patients dying before having a chance at a transplant.

However, this decision created a problem for Cameron and his mother—a purely financial one. There was the cost of moving to Pittsburgh, where they would have to stay until a donor could be found. Those costs were, however, meagre compared to the cost of the procedure and the subsequent post-operative stay in hospital, with ICU beds at that time running at a staggering $2,000US per day.

A fundraising campaign was initiated in his hometown. There were many who were inspired by this young man's positive attitude and his unflagging optimism. In the end, sufficient funds were raised, and he set off for his evaluation. His assessment went very smoothly, and he returned to Toronto General full of enthusiasm. His positive attitude had if anything gained momentum.

"They are just wonderful down there. Doctor Todd, they are so understanding, I know it is going to work out great!"

Those were his last words to me before he left again for Pittsburgh. Several weeks later, we heard that his transplant had been successful. There had been significant post-operative hemorrhaging, necessitating a further urgent procedure; but he had rallied and was improving. It was arranged for him to return to Toronto General for convalescence before his discharge home, and I was eager to see him when he arrived on our ward. He was even thinner than I remembered, and although his infectious smile was ever present, the jauntiness was gone.Cameron had seen hell and, like the others before and after him, talked little of the experience.

As he gained in strength and was able to walk about the hospital without oxygen for the first time in several years, the bounce slowly returned and his animation and his joy at what appeared to be a huge success became evident. His happiness and relief were truly infectious, and I was pleased that we had decided to send him abroad for his operation.

But Cameron was to provide further lessons before the final chapter was written; a most important lesson that we as physicians continually relearn. There are problems that arise late and often they are created by the therapy itself. Rejection set in and another prolonged visit to Pittsburgh was necessary. Although that was ostensibly treated, he continued to fail, and we heard of yet another admission.

Then later in 1983 I ran into him quite by accident on our ward. Joel had been asked to take him back for a few days in transfer from Pittsburgh for another bout of convalescence before returning home. One day there he was, much like on our first encounter, strolling down the hallway pushing his metal IV pole ahead of him.

"Cameron, how are you? How did you get here?" I asked, slapping him on what were now very lean shoulders.

"Oh, hi, Doctor Todd—I'm here just for a few days to gain some strength before going home."

There was a quietness to him and an emptiness that made me want to put my arms around him and reassure him that all would be right. But then he smiled and said, "Are you guys ever going to start to do something and catch up to the Americans?"

Perhaps, I thought, he is still the same old Cameron. The moment passed; and besides, surgeons don't hug their patients.

He said, "Can you come into my room for a minute and look at my neck? I've got some lumps where they stuck the needles in to do the heart biopsy. Could you check it out?"

He was referring of course to the biopsy undertaken for rejection discussed above. The needle is inserted into the jugular vein in the neck in order to provide access for the biopsy catheter.

I did what he asked. The lumps to which he referred were indeed where it appeared they might have placed the needles to access the jugular vein. They were odd. I told him that it looked like a scar from the needle punctures. But there was an uneasiness in both of us—mine because I was not really sure. I knew they weren't scars; they looked more like a tumour growing there. As for his reaction, I don't know why he was so troubled. Perhaps he had asked the same question in Pittsburgh and received the same vague answer. It was the first time that I had waffled with him. He was a very intuitive young man.

As I left his room, for the first time since we had known each other neither of us could look the other in the eye. I saw him again two days later in the corridor during my routine rounds. He thanked me for what I had done on his behalf. I wished him well and we joked about Toronto trying to measure up to Pittsburgh. As I look back to that time, I sense how much had changed. There was a finality and a strain to our last conversation that had gone unacknowledged. We both I am sure recognized it at the time. I certainly see it now. That afternoon I did not realize it would be the last time that I would see Cameron. Perhaps that was the knowledge that had been left undefined. I think we both knew but were afraid to acknowledge the certainty of his end. It was certainly clear that things were not right and that his promise of a new life was unfulfilled.

Cameron died of a malignant lymphoma. It occurs as a complication of intense immunosuppression, particularly in young people. It is believed to be related to a certain viral infection and hence less common in adults who have already had the infection while possessed of normal immunity. It was lymphoma that I saw that day in his neck. Just before his death, his mother sent me a book at Cameron's request. In it he wrote, "On behalf of my mother and myself, this is a small way of saying thanks. Your support and enthusiasm has done so much for me. I honestly believe I have been in the best of hands." I felt that he had just expressed what I should have said to him, had I been granted the opportunity to speak with him again. His enthusiasm had taught me so much. I keep the book on my shelf for inspiration.

Linda was twenty-six and very frightened. Sensing death breathing down her neck, this mother of two young girls was unable to recognize her own strength. My initial and only pre-operative encounter with her was the antithesis of my meeting with Cameron Evans. It was late and I had just finished an emergency operation. Knowing that the next day would be no better than this one, I decided to stop in to see her before going home. There had been some urgency in this consult request and again I was late. The hospital corridors had been darkened down for the night, visiting hours were over, and the place had the solitude that always pervades the off-hours in a hospital. That's probably why I could hear her crying in the dark before I even entered the room.

Her medical problem was the same as Cameron's— pulmonary hypertension. Nonetheless, the progression of her disease had been especially rapid and she was now bedridden. As a result, the team had accelerated her assessment. The reluctance and the tardiness that the program had assumed following Jack's death had seemed to evaporate. This girl was going to receive a transplant, I had been told. Walking over to the College wing to see her that night, I had to wonder if the urgency was due to the condition of the patient or that of the program.

Our interview was too brief and too lacking in substance. She did not hear or understand the information that I had come to offer. She looked at me but all I could sense was the intense fear and trepidation that emanated from her like a current of static electricity that charged the air around us. The message I came to deliver went unheard and the optimism I wished to provide was unappreciated.

Physicians and patients often face a challenge when it comes to such communication. There is no doubt that many physicians are less than empathetic to their patients and frequently will speak in incomprehensible medical terms rather than take the time to explain the situation in a manner that the patient can fully understand. Whether because of their own discomfort or in ignorance of what is required, they do their patients little service. Likewise, however, there are patients who hear but do not listen. Not infrequently, patients are concerned that they will appear ignorant of medical matters and hence never ask for clarification. They merely nod in acquiescence. Sometimes, perhaps to quell their trepidation, their mind refuses to focus on what is being said. You can tell by the blank expressions on their faces.

On several occasions I have asked patients if they fully understood everything. After responding in the affirmative, I have asked them to tell me what it is they understand. To their own surprise, they simply cannot relate much at all and, embarrassed, ask for a repetition of the information. My conversation with Linda was like that. It was distressing because our impasse occurred in the midst of her intense inner suffering; she had already begun to grieve her own passing. She spoke of the distress her girls would feel after she was gone. There was just no response to my information. I was too tired to persist for long. Driving home that night I realized that she was likely correct. She was going to die. I became convinced that she should not be offered a transplant. The program could be ruined by another failure. The next day, however, it became clear that decisions had been made. There was no going back.

Several nights later, a donor was found and flown to Toronto. It was April 22, 1983, three days after Linda's youngest child's first birthday. The excitement was still there in the operating room that night, but I could sense that Joel also was having misgivings. It just didn't seem right. Things had gone too fast and we were too unsure of this patient.

But as we stood at the scrub sink discussing the sequence of the procedure, the adrenalin rush returned, and entering the room I began to feel confident and that my fears were merely the result of the young woman's obvious distress that night. To solidify that resolve, the donor lung arrived in the operating room in excellent condition. The case went very smoothly. As per our protocol, the anaesthetist stayed with Linda in the operating room for about forty minutes after we were finished to ensure perfect stability before transferring her to the ICU. Throughout that time she was stable—there were no problems. Later, I would review the entire operating record in minute detail and find nothing amiss, no hint of an impending problem.

I returned to the ICU for some much-needed caffeine. We had started the operation at 0300 hours and it was now noon. A long day still loomed ahead. One of the nurses strolled into the lounge and commented that they had just brought Linda into the unit from the operating room.

"Everything okay?" I asked.

"As far as I know. They're just getting things set up in there."

I gulped the remnants of my coffee and walked down the hall to the room that had been prepared for her ahead of time. She was alone in the three-bed room in the corner of the unit. We employed this room for transplant patients and ECMO runs because of its size, even though we lost two beds to the overall complement. Jack Collins had spent a long time there. Donning my hat and mask, I walked in.

"How's it going?" I asked.

Wilfred Demajo, who had given a perfect anaesthetic, muttered something that I never did catch, but took as promising. The nurses were busy with the intravenous and monitoring lines, which were tangled in a spider web of plastic. They were beginning to convert from the operating room monitoring system to that in the ICU. I watched as they calibrated the transducers. I always hated this time during a transfer when there was no data to deal with; nothing to reassure me that everything was as it should be. I wished I had stayed in the coffee room. Just then, though, they flipped the switch to link the transducer with the monitor, and the characteristic wave pattern of the blood pressure appeared across the screen. Except that it was blunted. It looked dampened as if the entire electrical signal was not recorded. As a result the digital read-out of her blood pressure was also low. In 1983, we were still using water-filled transducers rather than solid state. Thus, not infrequently, air in the system would distort the pressure wave. I wasn't concerned yet.

"Flush the line," I requested. Such should eliminate any air in the transducer and provide a more representative tracing.

They did, and the wave appeared much the same. The digital reading was, however, even lower. Now I was concerned. I began to realize that perhaps this pressure record was actually correct.

"Check it with a blood pressure cuff," I asked somewhat too loudly.

I could see the concern mirrored in the faces of the nurses. Now there was heightened activity, and a sense that something was wrong. I heard one of the nurses speak into the intercom.

"I think we need more help in here."

Wilfred looked across the bed at me. "She was okay, Tom. Her pressure was fine; there were no problems."

"I know, Wilf, but look at that." I pointed at the monitor. Her pressure was continuing to slip. It was now ten minutes after twelve and it was extremely low. Quickly I assessed the amount of blood in the chest drains, recognizing that bleeding would be the commonest reason for what we were witnessing. I ran to the other side of the bed to check her preload. This is the pressure in the veins as they enter the heart and is an index of whether the patient has sufficient blood in his or her system. It was normal, suggesting that she was not bleeding. I shouted to the nurses to get me some calcium and to hang some dopamine (a drug like adrenalin that drives the heart and artificially increases blood pressure). Two other nurses scurried into the room. The alarm was general now, and there were faces pressed against the glass window that looked onto the corridor. As usual, Wilfred was ahead of me as he gave her a shot of neosynephrine (a drug like adrenalin) from a preloaded syringe in his pocket.

"Always prepared" he said grimly.

I followed him with some calcium and her pressure began to improve. Within a couple of minutes, it was in the normal range. I quickly again checked the chest drains that came from her chest to ensure that there was no excess bleeding. Only a small amount was apparent. The nurses hurried to complete all the calibrations and to sort out the ventilator tubing and monitors. I drew a blood gas analysis from the radial artery line to check her oxygenation and carbon dioxide levels. It was processed immediately in the stat lab adjacent the ICU. I was very uneasy. She looked pale and her nail beds were dusky. I had the result in minutes. Viewing the numbers I knew our troubles had only just begun. Her haemoglobin (the measure of red blood cells in her system) was, however, normal, again suggesting that she was not bleeding.

As quickly as it had come back, her blood pressure disappeared. Now there was palpable panic as the nurse shouted that she could not get her pressure with a blood pressure cuff either. Another shot of neosynephrine from Wilf brought virtually no response. By 1220 we were in full arrest and cardiopulmonary resuscitation was commenced.

"Call Joel, he's in his office!" I shouted to Carol, the head nurse, who was standing at the doorway directing traffic. In the same breath I asked for a thoracotomy set to open the chest. It was clear that I was going to lose her shortly and I did not know why. We had pumped her full of drugs and fluids. There was nothing further to do but open her chest right there in the bed in the hopes that there was some surgical misadventure that was correctable. I could at least provide open cardiac massage. The chest opening was quite straightforward as the incision was already there. After opening the skin incision I merely had to cut the wire sutures approximating the two halves of the sternum (breast bone) and there was the heart. It was 1230 with Joel steaming into the room as I grasped her heart and commenced the rhythmical massage. The heart was full of blood as it should have been and there was no blood accumulated in the chest. Thus it was immediately clear that she had not been bleeding. Although that would have implied a surgical mistake, I had hoped that I would find something that easy to correct.

As I compressed her heart, her pressure rose but never approached the values we needed, nor did her heart acquire a spontaneously normal rhythm. We quickly reviewed all the options. What stone had we left unturned? What had we missed in all this? A few more drugs were given. Defibrillation of the heart was undertaken repeatedly as she oscillated between ventricular fibrillation and asystole (no heart beat at all). We extended the incision to provide a more generous assessment of the chest and the transplanted lung so we could more minutely examine the anastomoses. But nothing restored her blood pressure. We began to respond to the varying cardiac rhythms automatically; silent pauses replaced the din of the initial turmoil.

"It's been forty minutes now with nothing," someone bravely muttered.

"Wilf, Joel, what do you think?" I asked, deftly sharing the guilt I felt. I did not want to assume the sole responsibility for abandoning our efforts.

Sixty-five minutes after returning to the ICU, we ceased our efforts.

The nurses worked quietly to clean the patient for the family. We said not a word to each other as we closed the incision, paying no attention to the normal layers, feeling less like surgeons and more like proctors in the autopsy suite. The noise from the hall had ceased, and Carol had removed the faces from the window. As I closed this incision for the last time, I caught her eye over Joel's shoulder. She sympathetically shook her head and pointed to the waiting room reminding me that the next major challenge of the day awaited us shortly. The nurses spoke only the essentials—a request for this, a question about that. It was the typical silence that follows an unsuccessful resuscitation. The chatter would come later, the exaggerations developed, the armchair comments made. We would echo, "If only we had . . ." And "If it hadn't been for . . ." But for now, it would be quiet. It didn't matter anyway, as nothing could alter the brutal reality of this sudden death. Linda had known it all along.

It had been a long and tumultuous year. We had transplanted two individuals three times without achieving our goal.Cameron had gone elsewhere for his procedure and, despite our best efforts to find him peace, he also had succumbed in the post-operative period. We had of course been busy doing all the other things that characterized an academic thoracic surgical practice. Although the transplants were extremely time intensive, in reality the program had occupied a fraction of our professional time over the year. We all quickly retreated to those areas where achievements occurred regularly.

For Joel, whose prime concern was the program, it was more difficult. Yet he kept the idea alive and continued to analyze the reasons for our failure. Thus he came to the conclusion that our failure after all our cautious preparation had been due to our ready acceptance of patients whose disease had taken them too far along the natural course to be retrieved. We would no longer accept a patient who required a ventilator. We would avoid for now attempts on patients with pulmonary hypertension. In future, we would accept patients with pulmonary fibrosis who required constant oxygen, but who were otherwise stable with a normal heart. Patients with pulmonary hypertension, or those with infected lungs, such as patients with cystic fibrosis, would undergo heart/lung transplantation. Patients with emphysema previously considered appropriate for a single lung transplant would also be offered heart/lung replacement. We were shifting gears and adopting heart/lung transplantation as an adjunct to the program.

To many of us this seemed as if the end of the original objective had arrived. Only one entity that resulted in respiratory failure would remain as a possibility for the single lung program—pulmonary fibrosis. All others would be offered heart/lung as an alternative. Yet we remained convinced that isolated lung transplantation could be accomplished and that it would provide an option that in the end would be superior to heart/lung. A single lung program could offer two lungs and a heart from a single donor, thus providing a lifesaving procedure for three patients. This was considered an important objective when up to fifty percent of patients died on the waiting list for an organ. It could also avoid the rigours of cardio-pulmonary bypass, which was a prerequisite for a heart/lung procedure. Joel knew this as well, but his was the position of leadership; on his shoulders lay the responsibility of protecting the program from its detractors. Simply put, the program needed a success, and as heart/lung transplantation was already a reality, that seemed a good place to which we might direct our retreat.

In 1983, the heart/lung programs had reached the pinnacle of acceptance within the medical community. The rivalry between the heart/lung programs and our fledgling attempts at lung transplantation was intense, fuelled to some extent by the egos of competing academic centres. We were thoracic surgeons. The heart/lung programs were under the auspices of cardiac programs. Thoracic surgeons who concentrated on non-cardiac issues were unusual in those days, and Toronto was considered the main training centre for Americans, given the paucity of such concentrated thoracic activity in that country.

In the USA—in most countries—the specialty of cardiothoracic surgery was pre-eminent, although historically it had been referred to as thoracic surgery before the explosion of cardiac surgery in the latter half of the twentieth century. With the advent of bypass surgery in the 1970s, most chest surgeons concentrated their activity in the cardiac sphere and pulmonary surgery took a back seat. Pulmonary disease received little scrutiny from these surgeons. The operative cases were frequently relegated to the end of the day's surgery. The advances and technical expertise in non-cardiac thoracic surgery began to fade in such centres.

Yet in Canada, and particularly in Toronto, two divisions of surgical activity emerged—those performing cardiac and vascular cases and those undertaking the remainder of the surgical pathology in the chest. The rivalry between the cardiothoracic and the thoracic surgeons was intensified when isolated pulmonary transplantation was again attempted in Toronto, it having failed so miserably in the past. Stanford, Pittsburgh, and even London, Ontario (a mere two-hour drive from Toronto), had initiated heart/lung transplant programs and were reporting success. It thus became clear that if we were to be seriously considered as a thoracic transplant centre, we would have to hop aboard that train—at least for awhile. In doing so, we recognized that the transplantation of the heart and the lungs together had largely been undertaken for cardiac problems, usually for forms of congenital cardiac disease where the lungs had been irreversibly damaged from the primary cardiac cause.

To perform this operation just for lung disease presented some peculiar problems that all the above centres had encountered. Basically, the replacement of the heart and the lungs is a technically straightforward operation. As I have noted, it is much simpler than a single lung transplant.

Heart/lung transplantation also requires cardio-pulmonary bypass. A prerequisite of bypass is anticoagulation, as it clearly would be disastrous if there were clotting of blood in the external circuitry. That usually does not represent a problem if the surgical area is small and easily controlled. Nonetheless, even after routine cardiac bypass, a number of patients are returned the same day for further surgery because of ongoing hemorrhage. Patients with lung disease frequently have dense adhesions between the lungs and the inside of the chest cavity. These result either from inflammation due to infections or, sometimes, from previous surgery. Adhesions are not just tedious to divide in order to remove the lung but they are often extremely vascular. Thus, as we divide the adhesions, we also cut across a myriad of tiny blood vessels that readily bleed. The entire surface of the lung may be covered by such adhesions.

You have likely experienced the difficulty in stopping the constant ooze of bloody fluid from a deep scrape when someone has been injured. Imagine then the problem with blood loss from the entire inside circumference of your chest cavity following the division of all these adhesions, and then magnify that with the anticoagulation required for heart-lung bypass. Basically, it sets the stage for significant intra-operative as well as post-operative hemorrhage. In cases of cystic fibrosis and other types of infectious lung disease, this resulted in the frequent return of the patient to the operating room because of continued bleeding.

One of the touted advantages of heart/lung transplantation was the fact that the biopsies for monitoring rejection could be easily performed. I noted such when relating the course of Cameron Evans. In 1983, we were beginning to wonder if the heart and the lung could reject independently of one another, such that the cardiac biopsy might appear normal when indeed the lungs were rejecting. Those observations were formally published in 1986. This concern seemed to constitute yet another valid reason not to abandon isolated lung transplantation.

Last, and perhaps most important, it seemed ludicrous to replace the perfectly healthy heart of a patient with lung disease simply because the technical parts of the operation were more straightforward. Why provide another organ for possible rejection? As already noted, this argument gains even further momentum when one considers the scarcity of available donors. If the heart were not an essential ingredient, then it could be used for another patient anxiously awaiting a donor. This became a telling argument, in that heart transplantation had become highly developed, with significant long-term success. In addition, one could envisage in 1983 what would become reality by the end of the decade—that a single donor could supply thoracic organs (a heart and two lungs) to three separate patients. Thus, one had to ask the ethical question: "Should a donor supply a heart/lung when only the lung is required and the heart and one of the lungs could be used elsewhere?" This became an important question for a physician who watches up to thirty percent or more of his patients die on the waiting list for lack of an appropriate donor.

This discussion goes on today, although for somewhat different reasons. We now know that the exercise tolerance and functional reserve of a patient who has received two lungs is superior to one who has undergone a single lung transplant. Thus, the patients themselves clearly would prefer to undergo a double lung procedure. This of course denies the program the ability to provide a lung to another recipient. There are some patients who, because of their specific condition, must receive two lungs. But for those for whom a single lung is satisfactory the debate rages—do we provide superior lung function and long-term stability to fewer patients or provide the opportunity for prolonged life to more individuals?

In the summer of 1983, much of this was fire for a heated debate, a debate that took place in hospital lounges, in lecture halls, and on international podiums. All the facts were unknown, even though pearls of truth were beginning to sprout forth. This would all be important for the future, but at the time our concern was with a failing program that ran the risk of annihilation. Thus, heart/lung transplantation, or—as Joel euphemistically referred to it—lung/heart transplantation was incorporated into our program. For many of us, the reversal of the names was little consolation for the disappointment we all felt. Nonetheless, a measure of success would be required if we were to continue.

CHAPTER 5

Diane

I had never felt any ownership of the heart/lung program. Perhaps that is why I continue to refer to it as heart/lung rather than lung/heart, as Joel would have preferred, in an effort to emphasize our primary focus. But in reality, I am sure it was simply because it had been developed elsewhere. We were simply copying others, and I was perfectly aware that despite protestations to the contrary, it was indeed an admission of failure.

At first I was concerned that we might never attempt another isolated lung procedure. If it had not been for the wonderful rapport we had developed with those initial patients, and the great sense of responsibility that we all felt towards their successful completion of the transplant process, perhaps that might actually have happened. There was certainly one very positive aspect to the incorporation of lung/heart transplantation into the program. Once the announcement was made, the number of potential recipients increased dramatically. Even the patients themselves seemed to be sending us a subtle message that our time had not yet arrived.

Into all this walked Diane Hiebert. She was from Quebec and had been waiting on the Stanford transplant list for some two years. She was small or, more fitting—given her French ancestry—petite. As a result, finding a donor that would provide sufficiently small organs to fit comfortably into the rigid box created by a small rib cage had been a daunting task. Diane had watched her compatriots on the Stanford waiting list proceed ahead of her to successful transplantation simply because there was never a donor that was of the correct size. Many of these had joined the program long after she had. In Toronto, she would be one of only a very few on the waiting list of a program eagerly anticipating its first success. After weighing the odds of waiting for a donor in the USA versus one in Canada, she opted to join the Toronto program.

She was clearly a survivor. You could see it in her bearing and her approach to everything she did. She never expounded false optimism but rather exhibited a determination that was awesome and brooked no thought of failure. My wife would call her a pistol. Aggressive, inquisitive, she would attempt to direct the program more than function within it. Perhaps that was because she perceived it to be so immature when compared to the one at Stanford. We were small fry compared to them in terms of resources and organization. Indeed, they had originated the procedure and, as far as the transplantation of thoracic organs was concerned, had few rivals either in terms of their success rates or the contributions that they made to research in the area.

Diane arrived with a young daughter. Her male companion was a marvellous fellow who was intensely devoted to her. Even when the going got rough (and rough it was about to be), he was always there for her, full of optimism and support. He was a jewel who had stood by her throughout her long tenure in California and was her constant companion and supporter from the moment she set foot in Toronto General.

Despite the fact that she was one of very few patients awaiting the procedure, we, like Stanford, had initial difficulty in securing a donor of acceptable size. In the end, we determined that a compromise would have to be made if she were ever to be provided with the opportunity of transplantation. Thus it was that we transplanted Diane with organs that were just too large for her small thoracic cavity.

In Canada at the time, there was little competition for donor organs. We had a small program with few recipients. The corollary of this, however, was the fact that we witnessed several donors wasted due to the fact there was no "perfect match." Either because of blood type or the size of their lungs, the available donors frequently failed to be appropriate for those few recipients that we had anxiously waiting. It was a frustrating experience to frequently turn down a fully consented donor. It's hard for me to remember today why we chose that particular donor for Diane when the size of the organs was so discrepant. Certainly we had begun to feel that it would never get any better than this and that the risk of waiting for the right donor was greater than taking this chance. Suffice it to say that the donor organs were definitely too large.

If the organs are too large, then the pressure within the chest cavity rises, particularly when the lungs are inflated with positive pressure from the ventilator. If the increase in pressure within the chest is excessive, then the return of blood to the heart is impaired because of the pressure gradient itself. As a result, the volume of blood in the heart available for ejection decreases and the blood pressure falls. If the fall in blood pressure is significant, shock ensues and the tissues of the body do not receive sufficient oxygen and nutrients to meet their metabolic requirements. The natural history is of progressive organ failure and death.

This is the fate that awaited Diane as she returned to the ICU following what appeared to be an uncomplicated heart/lung transplant. The first few hours passed uneventfully, a stark contrast to the last transplant we had performed. As time passed, however, her blood pressure began to drift ever downward.

However, it is expected that the transplanted organs will accumulate fluid within them over the first few days due to the injury sustained from the extraction process itself. As noted before, the transplanted organs are bereft of an oxygenated blood supply for several hours. The effect is much like what you have observed after an injury. If I were to hit you over the arm with a baseball bat, the arm would swell and become tense, the skin would be stretched. The same is true of the lungs and as well the heart. In addition, as the lungs fill with fluid, they become more resistant to the ventilator's efforts to pump air. Thus to achieve the same volume of air for gas exchange, more pressure is required.

In the case of the thoracic cavity, the ability to stretch is limited by the rigidity of the rib cage. It simply doesn't stretch like skin. This problem, termed "reperfusion injury," was much more common in the 1980s, due to our imperfect mechanisms of preserving the extracted lungs. They were as a result more susceptible to the injury induced because of the extraction process and the fact that they resided outside the body for several hours. As Diane's new heart and lungs began to swell, the pressure in the thoracic cavity began to rise even more than it had from organs that were too large in the first place. This resulted in a steady decrease in blood pressure.

At the end of the first eight hours, we were concerned that the fall in blood pressure was secondary to blood accumulating around the heart and directly affecting the pumping action of that organ. This, too, was a recognized complication that can occur from any form of cardiac surgery, not just transplantation. In fact, although I have described for you the condition of rising intra-thoracic pressure due to swelling from the accumulation of fluid in the lungs, the entire phenomenon was not well recognized twenty years ago. Today the diagnosis would be considered at a much earlier stage, due to the accumulated experience that more frequent transplantation has provided. However, at that time, our presumptive diagnosis was accumulated blood compressing the heart.

As was our practice, we had provided for constant, dedicated, physician coverage in the room. That afternoon, the physician looking after Diane was informed of our concern. We noted that if the problem intensified, the only recourse would be to open the incision and evacuate what we presumed was clot compressing the heart.

The incision was similar to that performed for cardiac bypass surgery, involving a split of the entire sternum with the aid of an oscillating saw. The two halves are then wired back together. Opening the incision would involve cutting the wire sutures that were employed to bring the two sides of the divided sternum (breast bone) back together, much as I had done during the resuscitation of Linda months before.

The physician that afternoon was, however, not a surgeon. Ron Grossman was a respiratory physician from Mount Sinai hospital across the street. He was a strong supporter of our efforts and had volunteered to assist us with the post-operative babysitting. The thought of opening the incision in the bed, in the ICU, was a daunting proposition for him. It was fortunate for Diane that when it became apparent that it must be done he was able to do so. It was also early enough in the evening that several of us were still available in the hospital.

True to prediction, the emergency occurred. Ron acted boldly, based on what he had been told. Her blood pressure immediately began to rise as soon as he opened the incision. However, once I arrived and placed my hands in the incision it became evident that there was no blood around the heart causing compression. In addition, her blood pressure was again beginning to deteriorate. Visions of Linda danced depressingly through my head. We were in the same room and in the same precarious situation. Once again, the spectre of real failure loomed, and I was despondent. Ron, however, was euphoric.

"I did it, Tom. I opened her chest, me a non-surgeon. It worked! Look at her pressure—it's a lot better. Wow, that was amazing!"

There were other superlatives, but this captures the essence of his pleasure with himself. And why not—performing such an intervention in the bed is a significant undertaking for a surgeon, let alone someone who had never done it before. He was justified in his enthusiasm and in his relief that it had produced a positive effect.

"But Ron," I said, "the pressure is falling again. Are you sure you didn't remove clot?"

"There was blood, but I haven't done this before. How much do you mean?" he replied.

An examination of the bed and the hastily supplied drapes for signs of blood certainly suggested that clot accumulation had not been the problem. Still, the pressure required to ventilate the lungs had been rising while the blood pressure was progressively going in the opposite direction. Even now it was falling further, despite the fact that the sternum was now open. It was also apparent that the tissues in the chest, the heart, and the lungs were swollen. As the pressure continued to fall, Joel called over from the door, "Open the sternum further; spread the edges apart."

I did so simply by pulling on the edges of the bone itself. The blood pressure immediately began to rise. But as soon as I released my grip and the edges of the bone returned to their previous position it once again became quite unacceptable. Asking for a thoracotomy set that we had used when operating on Linda a few months earlier, I extracted a rib spreader. This is a metal retractor that enables one to spread the ribs apart when operating on the lungs or heart and hold them distant from one another. I placed the spreader between the two halves of the sternum and winched the sternum widely open. With the retractor fully open, her heart and lungs were exposed as if she were undergoing a formal operative procedure. In addition, the blood pressure suddenly improved to normal limits. It was now quite obvious that the problem was related to increased pressure in her chest. This was likely a combination effect from the insertion of excessively large organs and the resultant swelling that naturally occurs in all the tissues following surgery. It was simply too tight in her chest.

We stood there for the next thirty minutes waiting for some further deterioration to occur. There was no bleeding. No further decrease in blood pressure. She remained rock stable. The diagnosis was apparent and the corrective measures had been undertaken. We did, however have the not insignificant problem of a patient in whom the chest was fully spread apart, complicated by the fact that she was residing not in the sterile confines of an operating room but rather in a bed in a busy ICU. The situation was not as stable as it might appear to the unpracticed observer. The patient was stable for the moment, but the situation was precarious.

The longer the sternum remained open the greater the chances of internal infection or of infection within the sternal bone itself. The former would be a disaster in her current situation and the latter a major problem, given the fact that this complication of itself in a non-immuno-suppressed host carries a high mortality. Recognizing this, we made several attempts over the subsequent hours to decrease the distance that the edges of the bone were spread apart. All of this was to no avail. On each attempt, the blood pressure began to fall and we were forced to once again open the sternal spreader to nearly its maximum tolerance.

As the clock ticked, the swelling in her tissues, now fully exposed to the ambient air in the ICU, seemed to increase. Such of course would only magnify the problem. This was beyond anything any of us had experienced before. Recognizing that the swelling was likely to increase over the first forty-eight hours following surgery, we were committed to leaving the incision not only open but also fully retracted. One simply doesn't do that for days at a time. Such evokes the spectre of life-threatening infection, as noted above, which in a patient now receiving medication to suppress her normal immune function seemed certain to result in a fatal outcome.

There really seemed but one solution to the problem that might at least have practical merit. I don't recall whose bright idea it was to simply cover the entire chest in the sterile plastic adhesive drape that we routinely use in the operating room. It certainly wasn't mine—such a simple solution and one I must admit I did not think would be ultimately effective. The drape is made of semi-transparent plastic, much like the clinging material in which we wrap leftovers doomed to rot in our refrigerators. The only difference is the size and the fact that the underside has an adhesive manufactured into the material. The adhesive is very strong and sticks to skin, metal, and cloth. This type of drape is used to cover the exposed portion of the patient before an incision is made. It prevents the instruments and the surgeons' hands from touching exposed skin. Even though the skin has been cleansed with antiseptic solution, bacteria begin to grow on the skin, and the degree of potential contamination increases with time.

In Diane's case, the largest plastic drape we had in our operating room was placed across her chest to cover the defect in the sternum, as well as the metal rib spreader. It extended from her chin to upper abdomen, and laterally covered both of her breasts. Once in place, you could view the heart beating away through the translucent material. It was much like looking through a misty window into the chest.

Although a solution, it was not a happy one. In our distress, as we commiserated with each other, someone recognized the resemblance of the chest to the then popular alien in the movie *ET*. That comment provided the comic relief that was definitely required at that point. Diane will always be remembered in the ICU as "the ET girl."

As the days wore on, the ET simile provided progressively less levity. The threat of infection grew with time, but she remained very stable, with normal organ function. We could not, however, assess her neurological function. Indeed this had not been done since her surgery was completed, simply because we could not permit her to rouse, given the rather drastic measures we had undertaken to maintain her life. Thus she remained heavily sedated and paralyzed pharmacologically, just as Jack Collins had during his prolonged ECMO treatment.

I have often recalled the first time that I was faced with a similar emergency and had had to react like Ron had done. It was when I was a young intern on the cardiac service at the Toronto Western Hospital. The patient had undergone bypass surgery that day and was in the ICU, but not on a ventilator as Diane was in this case. In those days, the immediate post-operative patients occupied a four-bed room on the cardiac ward and the intern slept in the same room on a regular ICU stretcher. On nights when the unit was full, we got to sleep either in a chair in a small office across the hall or in another patient room.

In this case, post-operative bleeding had led to clot and liquid blood accumulating around the heart, placing pressure on the heart—so called cardiac tamponade. This results in a dramatic reduction in the amount of blood ejected from the heart, and shock results. This is what we had thought was affecting Diane. By the time I was alerted to the situation by the nurses, the patient was in a pre-arrest mode. The blood pressure was very low and the heart was slowing down. I opened the chest in the bed for the first time in my life, evacuating blood and clot and spilling it all over the bed, the floor, and myself.

I was vigorously massaging the heart when all at once it resumed normal contractile function and the blood pressure returned to normal. Suddenly the patient stirred and lifted his head to look straight at me, as I stood there frightened to death and holding his heart in my hand. I assure you that my own heart rate was about 140 per minute and urinary incontinence was not far off!

Nonetheless, I remember that in my panic I knew I had to appear calm and so I just said that all was well, that I was adjusting his drain and would he please put his head down. Fortunately, the anaesthetist had arrived for the arrest at that point and quickly sedated him.

With that incident in mind, we certainly did not want a repeat performance with Diane. Thus, she was kept heavily sedated.

The unit and indeed the whole hospital buzzed about "ET." There was a regular queue outside the window of her room, and we had to mount extra security to prevent too much of a sideshow atmosphere. There were many who asked for "just a peek" at this incredible sight. Just pull the sheets back for a moment, they pleaded. We did for some. It was just such an unusual and unique situation.

Joel's impatience finally got the best of him after three days. He was determined to close the incision in an effort to prevent life-threatening infection that admittedly might already be brewing. Diane was rolled down the hall to the operating room once again. The procedure would be performed under maximal sterility, which seemed somewhat excessively cautious after what had already transpired.

Disappointment, however, was to reign supreme in the operating room when multiple attempts to wire the edges of the sternum back together resulted in repeated and unacceptable decreases in her blood pressure. It was clear, however, that the fall was not as precipitous as it had been on the day of surgery. She tolerated the removal of the sternal retractor with the wound edges only three or four inches apart. The tissues appeared much less swollen. It was apparent that we were winning, but that Joel had arrived in the operating room a few days too early.

It was at this point that Joel in his brilliance came up with a unique and simple idea. While I was advising him to leave the sternum open and close the skin with a return to the operating room the following week for definitive closure of the bone, he came upon a means of providing complete closure of the bone that day. What he did only added to the legend that had already been established concerning this unique patient. Normal sternal closure involves the passage of a series of heavy wires around the two halves of the sternum and then twisting them together until the edges are solidly approximated. In Diane's case, Joel passed a metal rod under each wire after it had been twisted to approximate the bone so that the rod ran the entire length of the sternum. Another wire was then passed about the rod at its mid-point and brought out through the closed skin incision.

He worked quickly to set up the apparatus, as her blood pressure was dangerously low once the sternal edges were brought into proximity. Once the rod was in place and before we closed the skin and underlying tissues, Joel pulled hard on the wire around the rod, thus placing upward traction on the bone and distracting it from the heart underneath. Her blood pressure began to rise. It was clear that the heart welcomed the increased space, enabling it to fill more readily with blood and thus eject more with each beat. Her blood pressure remained stable, albeit somewhat lower than its normal value.

In the ICU, we attached the wire that was connected to the centre of the rod to a series of pulleys with a weight on the other end to provide the appropriate distraction. The entire effect was to stretch the muscles and the ligaments of the rib cage upwards with the sternum, providing for a temporary increase in the volume of the chest cavity.

In the unit, the entire situation seemed just too bizarre to produce a good and lasting result. Although there was admiration for Joel's ingenuity, I caught quiet snickers and outright critique that focused on the absurd interventions that the thoracic service would assume in order not to admit defeat. The patient's demise had already been assumed by many of our colleagues and nurses. Little did they understand that Joel was once again adhering to his oft-spoken philosophy of learning from the lessons of history. The apparatus was not unique, although the situation in which it was utilized was indeed a first. It had been described in slightly different terms by earlier surgeons for the management of chest injuries wherein multiple fractures of ribs led to instability of the chest wall and collapse of the lungs.

As the days wore on, the amount of required traction steadily decreased until the entire mechanism was discontinued. The wire around the rod was simply pulled out. Her blood pressure became independent of our interventions. The snickering and the criticism ceased. Like a hockey team whose fans have fallen off the bandwagon with adversity our popularity and support returned. No infection occurred. This was a truly miraculous outcome. Even standard uncomplicated procedures can result in a sternal wound infection. Cardio-thoracic surgeons are meticulous to the point of being both anal and paranoid in their attempts to prevent this disastrous complication. Any break in sterile technique fills their hearts with dread and they wait with anxious anticipation for the days to pass until the fear of infection can be safely overcome with the passage of time. There certainly was a break in sterile technique here—for three days, no less! Add to this the fact that the patient was immuno-suppressed and hence even more susceptible to infection, and the wonder of it all was even more impressive. Diane's incision healed perfectly and she improved daily. She was weaned from the ventilator and returned to the ward.

Diane survived and spent many years as an advocate for the transplant movement in her native Quebec. Her legend has lived on in her own personal achievements. She established a foundation for the support of transplant patients and her name is synonymous with transplantation in her province.

But the uniqueness of her course in hospital was yet to be over, despite the fact that her subsequent medical course was largely uneventful. She did experience what we would later come to realize were quite routine episodes of early rejection, but they were readily treated. Thus the unique episode that follows was not entirely of a medical nature.

Just prior to her discharge, I was making rounds with the residents and the evening nursing staff at the end of the day. Diane's room was the last on the circuit, a private room adjacent to the nursing station. After reviewing her medical condition and sorting out with her what was now really just maintenance management (things that today are handled as an outpatient), she asked if she could speak to me alone. The request was not at all unusual for Diane, as she was an extremely assertive individual who made every effort to direct her own medical care. Indeed, this is not an unusual practice for many patients who simply do not wish to discuss all their personal aspects of care in front of the entire medical team. Given the fact that rounds on Diane were always protracted, the others were pleased to have an excuse to vacate quickly and get back to all their other duties and leave me to fend for myself. Once we were alone, she turned to me and asked: "Dr. Todd, can we have sex?"

Being an egotistical fellow, I of course assumed that the "we" meant she and I. Instead of being debonair, aloof, and complimented, I immediately flushed, became extremely uncomfortable, and uttered an incomprehensible stuttering of lord knows what. She immediately recognized my misunderstanding by this sudden change in my demeanour.

"I don't mean you and me! I mean my partner and I! Am I well enough in your opinion for us to have sex?" she said.

"Well, sure you are . . . there should be no problem," I replied with quick relief, flustered by my own stupidity.

"Good. Then do you mind if we do it tonight?" she replied.

"You mean here in the hospital?" I said incredulously, as once again I was totally off balance.

"Sure, why not? This is a private room. We're not going to disturb anyone."

Remembering her near brush with death and the restrictions—including those of the flesh—that had been placed upon her for several years, it was hard to deny her this undertaking. I certainly did not want to appear unenlightened after already appearing somewhat unworldly. As well, I had learned from these unfortunate patients that it was their appreciation of, and their zest for, life that sustained them through the dark times they all experienced. So I replied: "Diane,

I don't care what you do with the door closed. Medically you're fit and well enough. Just don't advertise it. Keep it discreet."

She was profuse in her gratitude.

When I returned to the nursing station, I began to appreciate the situation in a little more depth. What if a nurse were to stroll in there in the heat of the moment? I would certainly look a little ridiculous when Diane indicated that I had sanctioned the event. With as much discretion as possible, I spoke to the charge nurse.

"Look . . . later tonight, Diane and her partner may become sexually embroiled (I can't remember how delicately the wording went). If the door is closed tight—just stay away. You know she's basically well enough to go home. Ignore any activity there."

To my delight, although she was somewhat astonished at what I had to say, the nurse in charge raised no objections. But that would not be the end of it. With time to contemplate the matter, the nurses would make me wish that I had kept it a secret. Later that night, a frustrated chief resident called me at home. The nursing staff was now very uncomfortable about this impending act of intimacy soon to be performed next to their station. They were concerned that should there be any biological effects from this unusual hospital undertaking, their complicity might be construed in a blameful way. They wished to be absolved of all responsibility and were demanding that we either forbid Diane this sanctioned activity or actually write an order in the chart that the patient could have sex.

Pausing at my end of the phone line, I was certain that there was no measure short of moving her to a ward bed that was going to stop the much-anticipated celebration she had waited for so long. Heedlessly, I told the resident that if the nurses persisted in their concerns, he should write the order. He did. To this day I am sure it is the only such order to grace a Toronto general chart, despite the many unique activities that have been undertaken at that institution. In the morning, I was welcomed by a very grateful patient and endured the stares and disbelief of the nursing staff while adjusting to the browbeaten, sullen posturing of my chief resident.

Diane was discharged a few days later. There was a press conference on the ward attended by her daughter and her partner. We were able to bask for the first time in the sun of achievement. Yet as we revelled in our apparent success, the latter was somewhat mitigated by the fact that we had not been the first or even the second to perform such a procedure with success. Indeed, this was a heart/lung transplant, not a lung transplant. The success was bittersweet in that it very clearly emphasized the fact that we had failed in isolated lung transplantation and that the prejudices of the other programs were justified now that our adoption of their procedure had immediately reversed our fortunes. Their prophecies of failure for isolated lung transplantation now assumed more substance even within the walls of Toronto General Hospital.

CHAPTER 6

The Dynamic Duo

After Diane was discharged from hospital, there followed a period of introspection and inactivity. We seemed to have entered a no man's land. We suffered from a lack of focus. Despite the fact that heart/lung transplant had been successfully completed and in somewhat spectacular fashion, there was nonetheless a degree of ambivalence apparent. On the one hand, we had accomplished the goal of a successful transplant. On the other, however, all we had really proved to the greater medical community and ourselves was that we could reproduce what others had already proven to be a feasible undertaking. In fact, it was argued within thoracic surgical circles, as well as in our own backyard, that we had capitulated in our pursuit of transplanting just the lungs.

There was thus an observable decrease in enthusiasm for the entire process amongst several members of the team. I included myself in their number. I began to pay more attention to the ICU and the developments in my own research laboratory than I did to the continued search for a solution to the problems we had experienced. A sense of deserved accomplishment still eluded us in the latter part of 1983. Despite a mental separation from the program, I still yearned for the big one—the uniqueness of doing something for the first time ever; a true isolated lung transplant.

The one thing that our recent success had acquired for us was a sufficient notoriety that patients began to be referred for consideration of transplantation. This vindicated Joel's decision to proceed with the heart/lung program. For the first time, we were able to develop a list of more than one patient. This brought its own series of difficulties. Criteria for selection had been controversial and problematic for our program in the past, and now it seemed to be insurmountable. The ideal patient to this point had to be someone who was sufficiently sick that an impossible solution seemed worthwhile to attempt. Yet he also had to be well enough that his dire condition itself did not preclude the outcome by making him overly susceptible to multiple complications.

Selection was a problem, but equal to that was the fatality rate of patients on the waiting lists in heart/lung programs in other centres. Several Canadians that had been waiting for considerable periods of time in the Stanford and Pittsburgh heart/lung programs began to inquire about acceptance into our program. This became of concern to those of us whose motivation for participation in the program was the desire to do "lung" transplants, not heart/lung procedures. It was apparent that if we did not accomplish our primary goal in short order, heart/lung would quickly overcome and smother our objectives. It would be difficult to deny them the donor in favour of the single lung recipient when the latter had yet to prove feasible.

Thus it was that I received more frequent requests from Joel to assess patients who had flown in from various parts of the country. They were to be considered for heart/lung transplantation. Those few that could have a single lung procedure were increasingly given to asking probing questions about the relevance and future of the lung program. One could not blame them. Nonetheless, the assessments became more tedious, and, as the summer of 1983 wore onwards, I became increasingly convinced that the whole concept of isolated lung transplantation was dying but no one was willing to make the proclamation.

It was fortunate, however, that our greatest protagonist, Joel Cooper, was quietly pursuing the goal with unrequited vigour. I was not even aware at that time that he continued on his own to solicit referrals for single lung transplantation. It should also have been obvious to the rest of us, as it was to him, that an increased referral base for all forms of thoracic transplantation would eventually turn up those who were appropriately suitable for lung transplant. He had made the personal decision to avoid desperate patients such as we had attempted in the past; patients who were *in extremis* at the time of acceptance into the program. He knew that we had perhaps one last chance to accomplish our goal. Thus the patient had to be perfect—not too sick, not too well. He or she could certainly not be on a ventilator and should not possess other systemic organ dysfunctions that would complicate the post-operative course.

Into all this strayed Tom Hall. A Toronto native suffering from pulmonary fibrosis, he did not present in dramatic fashion, as had the others who had so far appeared on our doorstep. Yet he fulfilled many of the prerequisites. He was continuously oxygen dependent, and was clearly approaching the terminal stages of his disease. None of the normal medications prescribed for his condition were making an impact on his symptoms or their rate of progression. He was acutely aware of his impending fate and was determined to make the most of his remaining time. He had in fact managed to travel from Toronto to the Atlantic for a last swim in the ocean he loved so dearly. He was accompanied of course by his omnipresent oxygen tanks and while swimming was attired much like a scuba diver but for a mere splash in the surf.

That trip alone revealed a great deal about the determination of the man and the singleness of purpose that drove him. In his desire to visit the Atlantic ocean one more time, he had called all through the northeastern United States determining where oxygen outlets were distributed, what their hours of operation were, and how he could obtain emergency service should he unavoidably run out of oxygen. He had rigged a bracket to the back of the front seat of his car so that he could carry several tanks at a time. He then calculated his own usage of oxygen and determined how long he could manage between each dispensing outlet. He then proceeded to weave his way, driving himself between Toronto and his selected splash in the surf. At night he would extend long lengths of oxygen tubing from his car across the walkway of his motel and into his room. He was fortunate that no one managed in the dark to stumble on the line and disconnect him from the gas that permitted him to breathe comfortably.

Tom was determined to make this last trip to the beach memorable. He was most anxious to dine aboard one of the ships anchored in the harbour, but found that the gangplank from the wharf to the ship was at a considerable incline, given that the ship was riding well below the level of the dock. He was certain that he could not negotiate that gangway after dinner. However, he was not one to be discouraged at a casual glance. Instead, he sent his family aboard so that they might determine if the ship would be even with the dock at high tide. Having ascertained that fact, he next checked the times of the tides. He ate on that ship as he had intended. He made sure that he arrived prior to the tide coming in so that he could walk down the gangway when he arrived. He then waited to leave until the tide had come in enabling him to walk out on an even keel. This was clearly a man capable of adapting his objectives to circumstance.

Tom's wife and family was also an important factor when he was considered for acceptance into the program. They were extremely supportive of him and recognized that the choices were his alone to make. Both he and they were obviously stable psychologically. They would be able to provide the necessary encouragement, enthusiasm, and understanding when crises ensued and when he lost his own drive and depression seemed to overwhelm him.

The post-operative period had become the roller coaster ride of the transplantation process. There were always to be episodes of rejection, pneumonia, respiratory failure, and various other infections and complications that would tax the resolve and the resource of any patient. The support of the family was seen as key to success. Indeed, it would soon be the case that when there was not a designated family member who would serve as a "support person," the patient would not be accepted as a potential recipient.

The support person was required to live in Toronto with the patient prior to the transplant and to be available twenty-four hours a day to the patient or the program. This was a major undertaking for a family. Often coming from outside Toronto, the patient and the support person had to provide for their own accommodation while they waited for a donor to be found. This could take up to two years! During that time, there were sessions of physiotherapy, exercise training, and various other appointments that occurred every week. The support person was to be there for each one, providing both physical and emotional assistance while he/she watched his/her loved one deteriorate as the wait lengthened out into months.

Each week, there was a support meeting chaired by one of our social workers. New potential recipients were introduced to the group, announcements were made, and problems addressed. Both patient and support person witnessed those who joined the program. There were those who were transplanted and ultimately left for home. There were as well those who died as an accepted potential recipient, never having received a chance at the operation they had waited for so patiently and for so long. The support group meetings would announce the death of recipients either post-operatively or while waiting on the list. The group would assist those yet to be transplanted to effectively deal with the loss of their newfound friends. Support was to become an integral part of our program—Tom's family was the first to teach us just how important this was.

But Tom had one major flaw. His white hair betrayed his fifty-nine years. He was almost a decade over the age that we considered to be acceptable in 1983. This made him appear less than ideal; I noted myself that it constituted an automatic dismissal of consideration. That was before I had met the man. In fact, Tom came to be considered quite by accident. His wife had joked with his chest physician at the Mount Sinai Hospital that it would be so wonderful if Tom could only be given a new lung. They had not appreciated the fact that the program was still operational. The chest physician responded that indeed they were still planning to make another attempt at the Toronto General Hospital. Tom asked for a referral.

Because of his age, his physician initially declined to make the call, but Tom continued to press the point. He had already come to the conclusion that not only was lung transplantation his only salvation, but that he was destined to become a world's first. He simply refused to accept the fact that we might refuse him and constantly demanded that his position be re-evaluated. As Tom himself stated, he could not believe that age was as important as motivation and confidence. He knew he would overcome the adversity of the procedure. He would become the first. He finally was given his chance.

Looking back over the years, it is humorous to note how much things have changed in such a short span of time. We were so concerned with Tom's fifty-nine years of age. Indeed, for many years thereafter, sixty was to be the absolute limit. It would remain the limit until 1995 when a sixty-three-year-old man threatened to take us to court if we failed to approve him on the grounds of age alone. Reluctantly and with considerable pressure from the administration of the hospital we placed that fellow on the list. He did get his chance at a transplant but died within three weeks of the surgery. Nonetheless, the age barrier had been broken and we were to continue to accept patients between the ages of sixty and seventy. In fact, we finally produced a paper that would report the excellent results of pulmonary transplantation in elderly patients. Seventy remains the age limit as I write this tonight, but I am sure that will all change within the next few years.

Tom was fully aware that his physicians were at the end of their therapeutic armamentarium. Yet one can imagine his ambivalence as he came to sign the consent form for the procedure. On the one hand, he knew that his demise was certain within the next twelve to eighteen months. On the other hand, if the transplant occurred before this arbitrary eighteen-month time frame, history would suggest that his lifespan would actually be *shortened* by undergoing the procedure. In addition, it was abundantly clear that his demise in the post-operative period would not necessarily be a quick and painless end. Rather it might well be a slow death as a result of the numerous potential complications that had to that point been associated with the operation. Jack Collins's post-operative course had graphically outlined that possibility.

Faced with Tom's determination and confidence in us, Joel was placed in a difficult position. We had strayed from our selection criteria before, only to be burned in the final analysis. To do so once again would definitely invite solid criticism from within the team itself, as well as from the international group of surgeons and physicians who were watching and waiting for our next improbable undertaking. There was little doubt that there were factions within and without the hospital who for a variety of reasons wished to see our project fail. But Tom was a man not to be denied, and Joel and the entire program quickly capitulated.

Tom did not have to worry about a waiting list for a single lung. By this time it had evaporated. He was the list for single lung transplantation. There were several awaiting lung/heart transplantation following our success with Diane, but Tom remained the sole person on his own private list (and in my mind the most important list of all). The whole issue was sufficiently sensitive that his acceptance was not made generally known. The call for a donor was made discreetly. There was little doubt that if his confidence in us were misplaced, the program would soon cease to exist.

Being a Toronto native, the first to become a potential recipient, Tom provided an enormous advantage to the program. Again we were to learn valuable lessons by accident and fate. Like all the others, he carried a pager so that he could be reached quickly should a donor become available. In that respect there was no difference. The difference lay in the fact that he could spend his waiting time in his own home, a familiar environment, surrounded and supported not just by the ubiquitous support person but also by his entire family and friends. His support system never changed when he became a transplant candidate. He avoided hospital admission and thus was not exposed to the highly resistant bacteria that unfortunately make the hospital and most particularly the ICU their home. He was industrious and exercised regularly, always pushing himself to the limits of his capacity.

It would be a while before this singular aspect of Tom's life became obvious to us and resulted in significant changes in our pre-operative program. Most breathless patients become sedentary. Not a surprising turn of events, considering that exercise of even a limited nature results in extreme discomfort. Breathlessness can often result in a sensation of impending death when it lasts for more than a few seconds. Recall if you can the air hunger, the rapid heaving of your chest as you struggled for air after a vigorous run when you were younger. It hurt. It seemed as if your lungs could not fill sufficiently with air and you took great gasps to relieve the anxiety. But it lasted only a short time. For patients with lung failure, this sensation lasts longer and occurs more readily because with minimal exercise, the saturation of oxygen in their blood stream actually falls dramatically low.

When an individual without lung disease becomes short of breath, oxygen levels remain satisfactory. The sensation of breathlessness is simply because your muscles cannot work any harder or your heart beat any faster to sustain the demands of your body for oxygen. Patients with limited lung function experience actual decreases in the saturation of oxygen in their bloodstream even at rest. With exercise, a further decrease occurs at a relatively early stage. In addition, their muscles are even weaker than yours, because they have become atrophic from lack of use. Their shortness of breath is truly frightening and it lasts for so long that with each episode they are never sure if it will recover; never certain that this is not the terminal event, that suffocation is not a few moments away. Given these sensations, it is certainly not surprising that they assume a sedentary existence, avoiding the stress that generates the problem in the first place.

The problem of course is that the proverbial vicious circle is established. As one exercises less, one's capacity decreases, the respiratory muscles weaken, and reserves decrease. We all understand that a lack of exercise results in a progressive decline in our tolerance for strenuous activity. Rarely do we consider the fact that complete inactivity will result in the inability to perform even the slightest exercise without shortness of breath due to the resultant muscular weakness and de-conditioning. Thus lung-damaged patients lose out on both accounts. Their lung disease results in a decrease in blood oxygen levels with the least of efforts and then as they weaken from lack of activity they do not have the muscle capacity to recover when the breathlessness occurs. As they become weaker, shortness of breath occurs more readily, not just because the lung disease has progressed but also due to the relentless deterioration in muscle strength and function.

Tom Hall truly loved life, and perhaps that is why he clung to it so desperately and refused to become another statistic. He received regular exercise and was permitted to live as normal a life as his oxygen tanks would permit. His penchant for exercise helped maintain his muscular power in reasonable condition.

Tom ascribed his optimism to the fact that he had been a salesman for most of his life. Clearly, however, there was much more to the man than that. The advantages that he enjoyed would become a routine part of the program in the future. The family as well as the patient would be carefully assessed. It would become a prerequisite of acceptance that the recipient and at least one family member take up residence in Toronto while a donor was awaited. This would permit adequate supervision of exercise and dietary programs. Patients would be required to regularly exercise on a treadmill with the aid of oxygen, something we had not previously considered. It hardly seemed feasible when the patient could barely move about the room. Although the requirement would initially appear so minimal as to not even fulfill the term "exercise," it permitted each patient to begin to use muscles ignored for several years. With time they increased their capacity. Their muscle mass increased, and, most surprisingly, oxygen requirements actually decreased as their strength and efficiency of breathing improved. We would be able to closely monitor a patient's exercise tolerance and be able to detect minor levels of deterioration while there was yet time to intervene and reverse the downhill spiral. A decrease in exercise capacity would occur before a detectable change at rest.

A family member (or a friend in some cases) would always be present to provide the emotional support and round-the-clock surveillance of activity that the program itself could not. Emotional support was a major aspect of pre-transplant care, for as the program grew, the medical staff would rapidly become less familiar with the personal needs of an individual patient. In addition, it was obvious that a family member spending every day with the potential recipient would be in a far better position to appreciate the toll that the anxiety of waiting exacted.

It was a mid-week evening in November, and Tom and his family were settling in for dinner when the telephone rang. It is hard to imagine the impact of such a moment. Hard to conceive of the emotional electricity that would permeate this family as he broke the news that a donor had been found—that tonight was to be the long-awaited night—the point of no return. Tom himself told me later that this was the only moment when he truly experienced doubt. He had talked about death with his family, and had come to peace with it himself. His affairs were in order, as he had resigned himself to the fact that one way or the other his life was entering its final stages.

Yet it is one thing to talk about death and quite another to stare it in the face—to reach this point of no return where the few words "I'll be there" likely mean you will never see the sun rise. You have with those words of acceptance consciously decided to risk your life on a chance where no chance has existed before. One moment earlier, you were about to ask, "What's for dinner?" and instead you are contemplating the fact that you may have already had your last meal with your family.

Dinner was to be replaced with anxious moments of packing and driving to the hospital as Tom reviewed a lifetime and made the most of the last few hours with his family. One might argue that surgical patients go through this process on a daily basis. Perhaps, but it is not quite like this. Other patients know that there is a risk, but very few know that in their particular case there has yet to be a single survivor—that no one has returned to the dinner table to enjoy even the casual conversation of a November evening.

So, what do you say when you are savouring the last private time together? How do you handle those last hours? Very few of us are granted the space, albeit small, when we can say all those things we thought of expressing but hadn't; or of doing the small acts of sympathy, gratitude, or simply re-affirmation of love. Whether you are the one to go or the one staying behind, it is that last and oft-missed opportunity to clear the slate, make good the promise, correct the wrong, or just simply express the feelings that we so often repress. Theirs was the chance to never regret in later years the reticence that such expression fosters; an opportunity to avoid being the one to say, "If only I had . . ."

"The lull before the storm" was often the way I would describe the drive to the hospital before a difficult case. Whether it was a trauma patient, a transplant, or a re-operation on a patient who had developed complications, it was a time when no one could bother you. Note the past tense, as now there are car phones and the lull can become just an extension of the storm. In 1983, it was a time to reflect on what we were going to do, to make a mental checklist; and once that was complete, to forget it all with the radio and the ball game or just to think about your last holiday and the coming weekend. It all is destroyed once you walk through the emergency door and take the private elevator to the second floor. There, at the heart of it all, pandemonium reigns. Everyone has his/her own unique message to relate to you.

"The donor's pressure is down—what do we do?" They've already been told. You're the third to be asked.

"Have you seen the x-ray? Are you concerned about the shadow in the left upper lobe?"

"I've tried calling the radiology technician five times—still no answer. Shall we call the staff guy at home?"

"Has a bronchoscopy been done?"

"Has anyone found Mr. Hall to get him in here?" He's just down the hall surrounded by about 100 onlookers.

"The admitting clerks are refusing admission because there are no beds."

"What did Joel say? . . . Are you sure?"

"Check these blood gases! They've got to be wrong—right?"

"Did anyone notify public relations?"

My wife says that I tune out at the drop of a hat. I've had lots of practice.

Everywhere there is activity as the donor and the recipient are prepared. There is a minimum of three donor surgical teams for one of these events, each after a different organ. The coordination of their tasks was a job left to Bob Ginsberg, another of my partners in 1983. This was not an enviable task. In point of fact, there is no one who has complete authority in directing these various individuals, all of whom have their own idea as to how and when things should be accomplished. The teams are often from different centres and, in North America, perhaps from both Canada and the United States.

Surgical personalities are somewhat given to aggressive behaviour, particularly when it comes to decisions of pre-eminence or the decision-making process itself. Surgeons like to be the decision-makers. They take direction about as well as a stampede of wildebeest. Each extraction team of course wants to be the first to proceed, and there was as a result considerable discussion at the scrub sink as to who had priority. Such efforts are today far more routine, as experience and time have managed to establish certain rules of engagement. Back then, however, the mere thought that a thoracic surgeon might want to include a small cuff of the left atrium in his extraction would send a cardiac surgeon into a virtual tantrum of shock and dismay. The whole concept of a discussion around the scrub sink is indeed an understatement of the true state of affairs. Coercion is a better term when applied to the winning side. Bob mastered it well—he was not nicknamed the "street fighter" for nothing.

I assisted Joel in the insertion of Tom's new lung. It was the fourth such procedure we had done together. It should have seemed routine by this time. Nonetheless there was as great a sense of excitement as there had been on the night we did Jack Collins's first lung. An overriding sense that the long wait was over pervaded the room and found expression in the attitude of every member of the team. We simply knew this was the moment we had waited for so long. This was definitely about to be a first. We were that confident. Tom was in better physical shape than any preceding recipient and his inner strength was enormous. I felt like a runner a few mere strides from the finish, knowing he had won the race and wanting to remember every detail.

The room we used that night was an old one that no longer exists at TGH. It was not the usual thoracic room. It had a gallery with a large window that looked into the room so that observers could pretend that they saw what was happening. "Pretend" is the correct term, as from the gallery you could see nothing but the backs of the surgeons, the green drapes covering the patient, the passage of instruments back and forth, and occasionally small snatches of the incision. As for seeing anything that was happening in the chest—definitely not. Nonetheless, it provided a good place for the entourage to sit and wait.

We began with Tom lying on his back while we made an incision in the abdomen from the end of the breastbone to just above the umbilicus (belly button). The omentum was mobilized through this incision and then placed in a pocket we had fashioned under the sternum so that it could be retrieved when the chest was opened. I remember that part quite well, as it was the portion that I performed myself, and although I had done it before, and although it was a simple portion of the procedure, I was nevertheless filled with concern that when we had the chest open we would not be able to retrieve the omentum when we needed it.

I remember that the procedure was somehow quiet. There was no tension in the room. People tend to talk a lot and talk loudly when they are excited and nervous. In retrospect, I realized how uptight we must have been during the other attempts. The change of amplitude in the room was remarkable. This was a time when every detail was memorable. For me it was such a magic moment. Many transplants later, those details are awash in a sea of recollections not all as pleasant as that night. It would as well be the last time that Joel and I would do this procedure together. Although we did not know it at the time, there would be forces that would change the complexion of the program and my own participation within it.

Tom received a single right lung transplant. It went smoothly. There were early anxious moments in the intensive care unit as I awaited the signs that would portend another episode such as we had experienced with Linda and Diane. But that soon passed as

Tom's vital signs remained rock stable. It seemed like any routine post-operative course. He was definitely quite slow to come out of the anesthetic, but soon he was obeying commands and co-operating with all the nursing staff.

As expected, he was ventilated with a mechanical respirator and thus could not at this stage communicate with us, given the presence of a plastic tube in his mouth. If you have ever received an anesthetic you will know that the period of waking is characterized by a sense of time lost and a disorientation as to place. Tom's first moments consisted of poking at his left wrist with his right hand—a movement that led to his being restrained, as it was interpreted as an attempt to pull out one of his intravenous lines. In fact, however, he was actually asking for the time, wondering how much time had elapsed since he had been wheeled down the corridor to the operating room. He was surprised to discover that he had lost thirty-six hours. He had been sedated after the anesthetic had worn off and his recall was non-existent.

Before recognizing that he was truly awake from the procedure, Tom, in his medication-induced haze, was convinced that he had died. He could hear his family talking through the post-anesthetic cloud, but he could not see them. He related to me subsequently that he remembered wondering if this is what death was all about: the ability to hear your loved ones about you, but without contact, either visual or tactile. Perhaps, he thought, you floated in a mist outside reality.

Such foggy thinking is reminiscent of near-death experiences related to an incredulous and questioning media by unfortunate souls who have readily accepted the altered consciousness of shock or even cardiac standstill as factual representation. Tom's experience was one of those. That he was indeed alive was made obvious the next morning. A friend and neighbour, who was in the coffee business distributing various types of coffee to institutions, had come by to visit. Unable to actually be admitted to the room, he had left his business card with the nurse. Nurses are very empathetic individuals. They constantly talk to the patients in the intensive care unit while carrying out their tasks. They realize that some of their conversation may get through to the heavily sedated form beside them. No matter how obtunded the patient may seem from drugs or head injuries, the nurses always warn them before undertaking any procedures. They tell them before they turn them, adjust their tubes, suction their mouths . . . and yes, they simply talk to them—at least the good ones do. They talk about the weather, what time of day it is, or what day it has become. In this case, the nurse dutifully spoke of the visit by Tom's neighbour, the man from the Gravel Coffee Company. She mentioned that she had his card for Tom.

Tom later said, "I knew right then that you could not get that in heaven, that he was not calling there. Therefore I had to be alive!"

After that, his mind cleared and he realized in no uncertain terms that he had made it through the surgery itself. The confidence and inner strength that he had displayed pre-operatively came bubbling to the surface as he fought to rid himself of the ventilator. I anxiously awaited the day that Tom would be taken off the machine and for the first time breathe spontaneously with his new lung. Although I knew that true success would not be realized until hospital discharge, the removal of ventilator support seemed the most important immediate milestone.

Jack Collins had managed only forty-eight hours of breathing on his own, and at that point we had become irrevocably stalled. Removing Tom from ventilatory support would be somewhat more troublesome. By the time we were ready to wean Jack from the ventilator—or should I say by the time he had sufficiently improved to permit us to think about it—he had already had a tracheotomy performed. Tom, however, was receiving his ventilator-driven breaths down an endotracheal tube inserted via his mouth into the trachea.

The re-instituting of ventilatory support, even for short periods, is easy when a tracheotomy is in place. You merely attach the tubing to the tracheostomy tube itself. As a result, the physician is more likely to re-establish support at an early stage. However, once the endotracheal tube is removed the re-establishment of ventilatory support involves the re-insertion of the endotracheal tube through the mouth. This involves some degree of expertise; an ICU physician or anesthesiologist must perform the procedure, and the patient is usually sedated. Paradoxically therefore, the patient is usually permitted to struggle for a longer period of time before the ventilatory support is re-established. This simply results in more fatigue and a patient in a much more serious state at the time that the physician provides for mechanical support again.

Given all this, one tends to be somewhat more cautious in the weaning process when an endotracheal tube is in place. Many ICU physicians will immediately deny that this is the case. However, the ICU literature speaks for itself. It has been repeatedly demonstrated that the time from initiation of weaning to complete withdrawal from support is much faster when a tracheotomy is in place. Certainly in Tom's case we did not want to remove the tube until we were certain that he was indeed ready—that his x-ray was clear and his breathing pattern normal. All that occurred on the fourth day—he seemed capable and ready for me to remove the tube. Later that day, however, he was to teach us another valuable lesson in respiratory physiology as applied to pulmonary transplantation.

I had removed the endotracheal tube when I was reasonably certain that ventilatory support would no longer be necessary. In fact I had delayed the decision for a full twenty-four hours, given all our previous difficulties. At the time, there was no question in my mind that he was more than ready. Nonetheless, within a few short hours, the nurses were calling to inform me that Tom was complaining of breathlessness. When I walked into the room it was obvious that he was distressed. He was visibly short of breath and actively complaining that he was unable to get an adequate intake of air. What was particularly impressive given his stoical behaviour was the fear that was evident on his face and the agitation in his voice and manner as he asked me to please re-insert the endotracheal tube. He actually wanted the ventilator back.

I obtained an immediate chest x-ray and arterial blood gases to measure his oxygen and carbon dioxide levels. I already knew from the oximeter on his finger that he had sufficient oxygen in his blood stream, which suggested that an immediate intervention was not necessary. I do not know what I expected to see when the results came back, but I do know how anxious I was as I waited. The last thing that I wanted to do was to wait too long and have a cardiac arrest on my hands before re-instituting ventilator therapy.

Whatever my assessment had determined, I was not prepared for an x-ray that looked pristine in combination with blood gases that were near perfect. The x-ray showed that his new lung appeared perfect and that the old fibrotic lung was shrivelled and collapsed, permitting the new one to expand even beyond what would normally be expected. In addition, the levels of carbon dioxide in his blood stream were too low, suggesting that he was over-breathing—hyperventilating. Oxygenation was terrific.

I was dumbfounded and unable to explain this event. Here I was with a patient who was convinced that he was about to take his last breath, and yet all my measurements suggested that he was doing just fine. In fact the data suggested an anxiety reaction. In addition, the patient was one we had come to know for his rock stable mood and stoical behaviour. Not one to panic, this fellow!

Hyperventilation, however, is commonly seen in anxious subjects. For a while I sat there wondering if Tom had finally become unglued, if I had overestimated his resiliency and resolve. He certainly, despite the fear that emanated from the man, appeared rational and amenable to a logical explanation. We explained to him that all was well, that there was no problem.

The new lung was in great shape, his oxygen levels were far better than they had been in many years. There was no cause for concern. I attempted to be as convincing as possible.

These assurances did little to alleviate his concern and his very visible, almost tangible anxiety. He continued to insist that things were far from right and that he was indeed in serious trouble. He repeatedly requested that I reinsert the endotracheal tube and once again provide mechanical assistance to his respirations. The entire scenario was improbable, for either this man was wholly out of character or indeed there was an unrecognized, unmeasured problem. No manner of reassurance was sufficient to assuage his concern. I began to worry and, as he told me that he sensed impending doom, I sensed my own rapidly approaching. I was in a Catch-22 situation. If I sedated and intubated him without a measurable cause then I would appear a buffoon the next day in front of my colleagues. On the other hand, if he was right and I delayed too long, a real disaster was about to descend on both of us.

I remembered the night so long ago when as a first-year resident in surgery I was called to the floor to reassure a young man in his early twenties. The unfortunate fellow in this incident had undergone removal of his gallbladder several days before and in fact was slated for discharge by his surgeon the next day. Despite all vital signs being impressively normal, the young man was convinced that he was about to die that very night. I did a complete physical examination. It was all normal. He literally begged me to help him. His fear was a wild thing. I even did an x-ray and some blood tests to reassure us both that all was well. I settled him down, went back to sleep, but was awakened three hours later to be informed of his cardiac arrest. He died that night of a pulmonary embolism (blood clot to his lungs). Yet there had been no physical sign of the impending catastrophe three hours before. But somehow he had known.

And so I sat with Tom for a long time. I repeated the blood gases several times and the chest x-ray one more time; more for my own reassurance and flagging confidence than for him. I attempted to provide a sense of calm for Tom, but I know now that my mere continued presence simply amplified his anxiety. In the end I came back to my resolve that Tom was a man of great inner strength and fortitude. If he was short of breath then there was a problem—it could not just be apprehension on his part. He certainly had the perception of breathlessness. For the first time it occurred to me that perhaps we had found the right word—*perception*. He had the *sensation* of breathlessness. There was no physical problem.

I recalled an article written several years before, describing the pulmonary function and breathing pattern of patients recovering from severe lung injury months after their apparent recovery and discharge from hospital. The author described patients who had retained a sense of shortness of breath and were found to be mildly hyperventilating when all other parameters of lung function had returned to normal. These two facts suddenly began to come together to reveal what may have been the truth behind the problem. Tom's problem was that he still had two lungs; one newly transplanted lung and his old fibrotic and partially collapsed one. The new one was denervated by virtue of the fact that to remove it from the donor all the nerves had to be severed. He had no sensation from that lung! The old one, however, had all its nerves intact. We know that the lung has a variety of sensory nerves, one type of which is referred to as the stretch receptors. If the lung is not properly inflated, it sends a message to the brain: "We are short of breath down here! We need a good stretch— a good deep intake of air."

That is the mechanism behind yawning. In Tom's case the new lung was expanding just fine but the brain was entirely unaware of its movement. His old one, on the other hand, was stiff and scarred from his primary disease process. Expanding it was much like blowing up a balloon encased in cement. But it had a full complement of nerve endings. It was discharging its responsibilities by sending SOS signals to the respiratory centre in the brain. Because of this, Tom, I reasoned, had the perception of breathlessness, when in reality all was normal.

Now this was merely a hypothesis and still is today very difficult to prove, but it seemed to fit what we were witnessing. I attempted to explain my thoughts to Tom. He was not easily convinced. Probably I didn't seem very sure of my newfound theory. I placed the oxygen saturation monitor on the bed in front of him. It gives a digital readout of the saturation of oxygen in the blood stream. Tom was able minute by minute to visually appreciate that his oxygen levels were perfectly satisfactory. I even removed his oxygen mask and for the first time in several years he was able to know with certainty that he could sustain his own oxygenation without supplemental support.

Simple reassurance had not been enough. Visual recognition of the facts, combined with a logical explanation that began to seem more plausible every time I said it, perhaps had a chance. He constantly watched the oxygen monitor. As the evening wore on the explanations began to have the desired effect and seemed to take root. His anxiety was alleviated. His hyperventilation persisted to some degree, but his confidence returned and both his and our distress lessened.

Later, Tom only vaguely recalled the episode. For me, however, it was one of those moments that begin with uncertainty and concern and finish with a sense of euphoria. A new dilemma never experienced before generates a new hypothesis that whether right or wrong satisfies the situation. We were to witness the situation again, and only in patients who had a single lung transplant where the remaining native lung was scarred and collapsed. It became my practice to forewarn this group of patients, and the foreknowledge appeared to minimize the subsequent problem. They were prepared for the unpleasant sensation and knew that it would be transient. Unlike Tom, they were prepared for the event before surgery and thus were disposed to believe that this was merely what we had warned them about before the operation. The mind is a wonderful thing and the problem has never been as acute. Mind you, we almost routinely now perform double lung transplants, so there is not much chance of observing it any longer. I only wish that I could know for sure if the hypothesis is correct; but I suspect I never will.

Over the subsequent two months, Tom rejected his new lung on two occasions, a pattern that was to repeat itself in most transplant patients thereafter. But in November 1983 we were unaware of the pattern and became concerned that the second episode portended graver problems. The first episode occurred following his transfer out of the unit and necessitated a return not only to the unit but also to the ventilator. He had been the first in our experience to manage an exit from the ICU, and his return was not well received. Once again, it seemed that we were to be knocked down just when success seemed evident. However, once again he rallied and was transferred out to the ward a second time; this time, we became somewhat less euphoric and suppressed our enthusiasm. Caution ruled the day.

We were to learn that optimism in this area did indeed need to be cautious. Never was this more evident than when he returned to the ICU for a third visit during his second experience with rejection. This time, however, we had intervened more quickly and were able to avoid institution of the mechanical ventilator, although it was the first and only time that Tom lost hope and his confidence faded. Even during the sensation of breathlessness following his initial release from the ventilator, he had still been confident of the outcome. But this time he felt his spirit slipping from him and if he could have willed his own death at that moment, there would have been no hesitation. He was just plain tired. Several years later, he expressed to me how he had felt at that time. I recorded his words that day, and what follows is a verbatim transcription.

"I was having such difficulty breathing and all you fellows were around my bed saying your counts look good, Tom. You are going to be all right. But I could still not get a real breath of air.

At that point my spirits went down. I gave up. Had there been a way of just dying at that point, I would have—if I could have controlled it. It was just such a disappointment after going through everything and you get that great lift and say By God! I have made it, I have lived. And then all of sudden you are back down. You are back where you started from.

"I now tell people that they are going to have emotions like a roller coaster. You will get tremendous highs and the next thing a tremendous low. When you get the lows you must remember that there is another high coming. That it is just a matter of living through the low periods. It is a terrible thing to face, especially after you have come through so much and you figure you have got it made."

Tom was the first to experience this and thankfully he had the fortitude to live that nightmare and emerge emotionally unscathed. I have too often witnessed the opposite. As physicians, we often fail to appreciate the importance of the patients' spirit, their inner will to continue despite the exaggerated fluctuations that can occur in their condition when they have a critical illness. I have seen it in their eyes—a helplessness and resignation that leads to an emotional withdrawal from all the events surrounding them. From that point onwards, they just fade away from us. No matter what we do, no matter what drugs we add to the armamentarium— nothing changes. They begin to slip away day after day unless you can get past their defences to the spirit and rejuvenate within it a sense of confidence that it is possible for them to survive if they will only give it one more shot. Tom gave it that one more chance and fortunately it was mostly uphill from then on. Another valuable lesson was learned.

Just as future recipients were to be prepared for the sensation of breathlessness after a single lung transplant, so, too, would they now be informed of the roller coaster ride of improvement, complications, and subsequent resolution. Tom's articulate descriptions of his experience resulted in the formal addition of a psychologist and a psychiatrist to the transplant team. They would participate in every phase of the program from pre-operative assessment to assistance in the management of post-operative depression and agitation, both of which became commonplace. They became an integral part of the entire recovery phase, providing insights and therapeutic options not obvious to a bunch of concrete-thinking surgeons.

Despite all he had taught us, Tom was to provide one additional insight before his discharge from the hospital. For nothing other than our own curiosity, we had decided to perform perfusion lung scans to determine how much of the cardiac output was going to each lung, native versus transplant. We had supposed that eventually the new lung would receive most of the blood flow—a good thing, since if there were significant persistent blood flow to the native lung, a large portion of the heart's output would not be properly oxygenated.

A perfusion scan is quite easy to perform. A radioactive isotope is injected into a vein and then the patient is basically placed under a giant gamma counter. The relative amount of blood flowing to each lung is thus determined by the concentration of radioactive counts over each side of the chest. As expected, we witnessed a progressive increase in the blood flow to the transplanted lung as the patient recovered from the surgery.

In retrospect in Tom's case, we noted that the perfusion to his transplanted lung had begun to fall just prior to both episodes of rejection. It then returned to baseline following successful treatment of the rejection. For the first time, this suggested a possible means of monitoring progress when a single lung transplant had been performed. Scans were instituted as a routine post-operative assessment. A decrease in blood flow to the transplanted lung indicated by the scan would suggest early rejection and prompt prophylactic therapy. Although we would in later years become more sophisticated in the monitoring of rejection, this was a valuable tool in the early years.

Once again, experience and accurate observation had shown the way. Looking back, it is evident that each recipient contributed in a very real sense to the development of the program. They contributed to our knowledge whether they died before we recognized the lesson learned, or whether they survived because the lesson was learned in sufficient time to assist in their success.

In Tom's case, success was indeed at hand. Certainly there were other setbacks, for the roller coaster ride is a lifelong game for us all. For some it is just more difficult and dramatic. He developed pneumonia in his native lung, requiring two weeks of antibiotic therapy. He was erroneously given a high dose of cyclosporin, the new immuno-suppressive agent—at least new at that time. The blood levels of the drug rose perilously high and we experienced several anxious days waiting for the toxic side effects to manifest themselves. Fortunately none were to come.

He underwent countless bronchoscopic examinations to reassure us that the bronchial suture line was healing appropriately. As the weeks went by and we waited for the proverbial other shoe to drop, there began a cautious optimism that the long wait was over—we had created something new. The day of his discharge, we had a party for him on the floor of the hospital—5th floor Norman Urquhart Wing. The press was invited and it was a joyous occasion. I have a picture taken that day of Tom and me together (Figure 7). When I look at it now and compare the image there to the man I would come to know over the next several years (Figure 8), I see the suffering expressed in those eyes and the incredible fatigue that was the result of all his efforts and our ministrations.

He returned to work a month after leaving hospital. We revelled in his success and his happiness. For the first time, a single lung transplant had resulted in complete recovery, not just survival. Yet none of us was fully aware at that time of the measure of this success. We were intent on the evaluation of the lung and had not as yet fully appreciated the measure of the

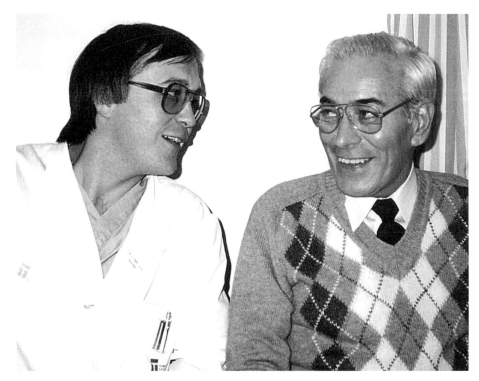

Figure 7. World's first successful single lung transplant recipient on the day of his discharge from Toronto General in 1983. Seated with the author.

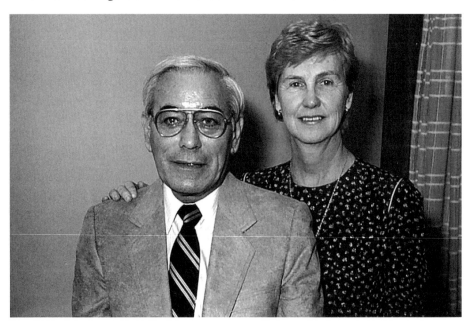

Figure 8. Tom Hall and wife, Barbara, years later.

man. For Tom proved to be a sensitive and articulate spokesman for the program. His wit and constant good humour endeared him to the press, other medical professionals, and, most important, the recipient waiting list. With his now publicized result, the list would grow from a single name to one that would soon be beyond our capacity. When asked one day how he felt having received a lung from a French Canadian, Tom quipped, "Well, now I am officially bilingual!"

We were to hold several symposia to relate the knowledge we had acquired and to describe the techniques we employed for donor and recipient operations. The initial session of the first of these was chaired by Tom Hall. He introduced the speakers and fielded the questions for them without introducing himself to the audience. When one of the members of the panel was asked just how functional the recipients really were, Tom picked that moment to dramatically step into the spotlight and introduce himself. He was a constant source of encouragement to others with terminal respiratory ailments. More than physicians, he was able to supply insight and advice. He received numerous calls from respiratory patients across the continent. Even when their situation appeared hopeless, and he himself was certain that our team would deny access to the program, he encouraged them to have their records sent to Joel or to have their physicians contact us directly. He always felt that a small morsel of hope provided a bright spot to their terminal months of life. Indeed, the wife of one such patient summed it up quite nicely. Her husband had been accepted into our program but succumbed in the early post-operative period. She said,

"Before his acceptance into the program, all we talked about was his death. What I should do afterwards. After he was entered on the list for a donor, the emphasis changed. It became . . . after my transplant we will travel there, etc." Although that patient never enjoyed the post-operative success of others, his last months were spent in anticipation rather than resignation. Tom provided these insights and the impetus for the dynamics of the process we had created.

Several years after his operation I asked him, "What was the biggest disappointment you experienced?"

To my surprise—and despite his evident good health—he said, "I always felt that the transplant would rejuvenate me. That I would feel like a thirty-five-year-old man again!"

However, he soon discovered that he possessed the lung of a sixteen-year-old in the milieu of a fifty-nine-year-old body. He was still a fifty-nine-year-old man and suffered all the same limitations. In the end, even a man with supreme confidence had to recognize certain restrictions. Nonetheless, at his fifth anniversary party he appeared as spirited and feisty as ever. I watched as the newsmen arranged for Tom and Joel to demonstrate the ability to breathe by blowing up balloons, while all the while he held centre stage, quipping and joking with those around him.

It was a great event, symbolized particularly by the gathering the anniversary provoked. In attendance were not just the members of the team but also a group of subsequent survivors of the procedure for which Tom was the pioneer. There were sufficient numbers that we could barely squeeze into a memorial photograph. In the centre of the picture is Tom, the Dean of the movement, a man very much at ease with himself. There at one end is Wendy, five weeks after her single lung transplant and ready to go home. Wendy had had pulmonary hypertension, like Linda, who six years previously had died within one hour of receiving her single lung. Without Tom and the enthusiasm and optimism he restored in the program, we would never have attempted another Linda. It had in fact taken us five years. Wendy was as much his success as ours.

In November of 1984 we tried again. It had been a year of mixed blessings. We had performed lung-heart transplantation with a modicum of success, but as I have noted before, that was not where our heart lay. Our single-lung recipient list, though growing, was in 1983/84 still small and the donors scarce.

Although we had achieved a world's first in pulmonary medicine and surgery, it was almost as if the thoracic world had looked at us and said, "Okay, granted that was pretty good, but can you actually do it again?"

Monica Assenheimer was her name. She, too, was Canadian. She and her husband ran a hardware store in a small town in Ontario. A victim of pulmonary fibrosis, she was not only oxygen-dependent but virtually reliant on a wheelchair to get from place to place. She had lost an incredible amount of weight and appeared withered and wraith-like (Figure 9). Visually she would have been convincing as a victim of Auschwitz or a patient with terminal cancer. Anyone who would not anticipate her impending demise had no eyes to see. Indeed, in today's program the woman would have been declined entry to the recipient list until her metabolic status had improved and she had gained weight. However, on a cold November evening we determined to settle the matter of beginners' luck.

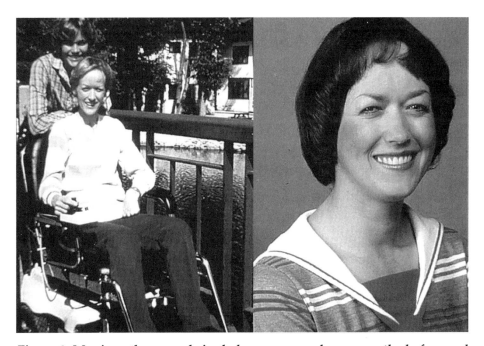

Figure 9. Monica—the second single lung success shown months before and two years after her transplant.

This was to be the first time that I left the recipient operating room to deal with the donor. It was with great reluctance. It was clear to us all that the rate-limiting step for the program was to be donor acquisition. We obviously could not afford to wait a full year between cases. It becomes somewhat difficult to maintain your surgical expertise with a particular procedure if you perform the operation but once annually. With each new potential recipient, we dreaded the inevitable question: "So how many of these procedures have you performed?"

Our response would hardly fill their minds with a sense of overwhelming confidence.

As intimated, I was to become involved with the donor side of the program. With donors, there were two specific problems to be addressed. The first concerned the assessment and the challenge of maintaining the donor's bodily functions until the point of surgery. Prior to 1984, the assessment process had taken close to fourteen hours before we could wheel the donor down the corridor to the operating room. That period of time was spent contacting the various transplant groups in North America to determine if they had a suitable recipient on their waiting list for one of the organs that this unfortunate patient was able to provide. Once contacted, there usually followed several subsequent calls before suitability could be determined. There was always an additional laboratory test that this particular program required. They had to find the right recipient. Then of course the donor team had to fly to Toronto. However, lungs are so incredibly fragile and susceptible to damage after the declaration of brain death, that this time frame proved very costly to our fledgling lung program. Most of the donor lungs became unacceptable by the time the donor operation was finally scheduled.

At Joel's suggestion, the surgical intensive care unit would take over the care of the donor. Our job was to streamline the procedure of assessment of donor organ function and to ensure that the donor lungs remained intact during that period. We were provided with a coordinator to assist us with the notification and organization of the other transplant teams. As director of the Surgical Intensive Unit, this responsibility fell squarely in my lap. Ever since my flight to Atlanta, I had been a member of the team evaluating the suitability of the donor lungs. Now that I would be responsible for maintaining the donor's lung function, it was a logical extension that I become the lead surgeon for the extraction procedure. Our senior partner had found the nighttime duty associated with this part of the program tedious and difficult, and we had a new and talented surgeon, Alec Patterson, to bring into the program to assist Joel. Nonetheless, it seemed like a demotion—the recipient side was the place of action.

The second issue revolved about the fact that we had insisted that lung donors be flown to Toronto. Our insistence had severely limited our access to the North American donor pool. Expansion of the program in Toronto demanded that we harvest donor lungs at distant sites. The development of this program was to be my other initiative.

Thus it is that my initial recollections of Monica's transplant revolve about an x-ray viewing box in the surgical ICU. I was assessing the chest x-ray of the potential donor who was resident in our unit. This donor appeared excellent. The chest x-ray was clear. The bronchoscopic examination was perfectly normal. Oxygenation was superb. But I could not resolve the problem facing me on that x-ray box. It was a two-panel viewer. On the left panel was Monica's chest film and on the right that of the donor. The discrepancy in *size* of the two lungs was not just notable, it was overwhelming. It was becoming increasingly difficult to imagine fitting the donor lung into Monica's diminutive chest cavity. I so indicated to Joel over the telephone.

Yet it seemed like such a waste of organs. Here was a great set of donor lungs. The donor was in my own hospital. It had been a year since Tom Hall's transplant. We seemed due. Looking back, I find it amazing to realize how limited one's horizons can be when you are locked into a singular mode of thinking. For some obscure reason, we had only considered doing a single right lung transplant, despite the fact that we had accomplished two, a right and a left, on Jack Collins.

The bronchus is anatomically more accessible on the right and the right lung is larger than the left, but otherwise I am now hard-pressed to remember why our approach was so rigidly defined. Nonetheless that was the case. On the right side, the liver sits just under the diaphragm and potentially limits its downward descent during the act of breathing. Indeed on most normal chest x-rays, the right diaphragm is higher than on the left side. On the left side there are only the spleen and the stomach, the former small and mobile and the latter easily compressible. It seems so simple now that it is embarrassing to note that at the time what followed in Monica's donor selection seemed like a revelation. As we sat discussing it on the telephone, neither of us able to dismiss this otherwise great donor, I said: "Look, we could go ahead with this, you know, if we just do the left lung instead of the right. That way the diaphragm should descend with the big lung and increase the space in the chest for the donor lung."

I went on to point out that the chest cavity of a patient with pulmonary fibrosis would always seem smaller than it really ought to be by virtue of the shrinkage of the lung that accompanies the disease process. There was a brief concern expressed that perhaps the left diaphragm might not work too efficiently if it was compressed downwards by the new lung. I was also reminded of the problems we had experienced with Diane Hiebert when organs that were overly large were placed in the rigid box that was the thoracic cavity. I argued that this time she would retain her own heart and that the native lung on the other side would likely collapse once a more compliant lung was transplanted, thus making room for the new lung. In the end, however, the best argument was the imperative of performing another transplant. A year was just too long between attempts. Joel agreed. We decided to proceed with a single left lung transplant.

After extracting the donor lung and delivering it to the recipient room, I left for some much-needed sleep. After all, I had been involved with the donor for several hours before the others had come to the hospital. As usual, I would take the first shift of supervising the patient when she returned to the intensive care unit. Thus a few hours' sleep would not only be welcome but essential.

When I returned to the operating room, Joel was gone. With the lung successfully implanted, he also had felt the sleep imperative and had been relieved by Bob Ginsberg. I found Bob and Alec Patterson quietly concentrating on this rather large lung bulging out of the incision between the ribs, and wondering whose bright idea had led them to a point where it seemed impossible to close the incision over the lung. It was obvious that the ribs would not come readily together without some major compression of this new lung. Ginsberg made the rather ludicrous suggestion that we now remove part of the precious lung.

At this point, as if he had been listening to us in his sleep, Joel returned to the operating room and abruptly vetoed that manoeuvre. As soon as he left, Bob did it anyway. It was clear that the donor lung was too large. The incision could not be properly closed. Thus a portion of the top of the transplanted lung was quickly excised with an automatic stapling device before Joel had an opportunity to return. I remain uncertain as to whether this made an appreciable difference to the outcome, but it sure made us feel better at the time. Despite the removal of the apex of the lung, the chest was closed with some continued difficulty. There were some sustained grunts and groans as Alex pushed the lung back into the chest while Bob sutured the ribs together.

I received Monica in the intensive care unit and concluded that the lung had adapted well to its cramped quarters. Her initial chest x-ray was excellent, but unfortunately, the radiographic appearance belied its subsequent function. Whereas

Tom's lung had functioned well from the start, Monica started off poorly and got worse. Naturally I immediately felt responsible. It had to be because the lung was too large. She not only required high levels of oxygen on the ventilator, but the x-ray picture, which had been initially clear, became cloudy and grossly abnormal within hours.

We presumed that the donor lung had not been properly preserved, although I personally continued to assume that the entire problem was size related. Whatever the reason, the new lung was clearly full of inflammatory fluid and was exchanging oxygen and carbon dioxide inefficiently. Although we administered diuretics to mobilize the edema fluid from her lungs and altered the ventilator settings, she became progressively worse. We undertook a bronchoscopy and cultured her secretions in the hopes that there was an unsuspected offending organism causing an early pneumonia. (Today we would recognize immediately that the problem was secondary to inadequate preservation.)

By the end of the third day, we had our usual meeting of the team in the coffee room of the intensive care unit. The possibility of a vascular complication was entertained. It was certainly conceivable that the veins or arteries had clotted or had become kinked, resulting in outflow obstruction of blood from the lung. Once raised as a possibility, it did seem to most of us to adequately explain the situation; and the fact that the lung had been shoe-horned into place suggested that such might have twisted or altered the normal alignment of the suture line.

Consequently, she was taken down to the radiology department for an urgent angiogram. An angiogram is an x-ray that outlines vessels. A radio-opaque substance is injected into the blood stream. The dye shows up within the blood vessels on the x-ray film and provides insights into patency and anatomical outline. Indeed, if taken in rapid sequence, as was the case here, the entire progression of the dye through the pulmonary artery into the lungs and then back to the heart via the pulmonary veins and left atrium can be visualized. The dye is injected through a catheter that is threaded from the internal jugular vein in the neck into the superior vena cava and finally through the right side of the heart into the pulmonary artery itself. A complicated procedure.

Yet the procedure is not nearly as complex as transporting such a critically ill patient on a ventilator with multiple life-sustaining drugs and attached equipment and monitors down a corridor into an elevator, down one floor, and along another set of corridors to the room where the procedure is to be performed. To do so, one basically moves the intensive care unit with the patient. A nurse, a respiratory technologist to assist with the machines, a doctor, and an orderly provide the motor power for the hospital bed, while watching the intravenous lines, various pumps, and monitors. One also manages to provide breaths for the patient with a portable bag and hopes that it adequately replaces the ventilator, which is now from a functional point of view a world away.

Monica's condition was critical and the decision to move her to the radiology suite was not made lightly. Of course, after all that effort the films reported that all the vascular anastomoses were intact and patent. Obstruction of blood flow was not the problem.

We met again, and again I felt that sinking sensation that the entire problem was related to the crowding of the donor lung in a chest for which it was never intended. If that were the case, then my responsibility became quite evident. Although most of our decisions were made by consensus, this one had clearly been pushed ahead by myself, and it was more than evident that several members of the team had had reservations from the very beginning.

We had never (nor do we now) spared criticism of each other. I believe that's a defining characteristic of most innovative surgical programs. From the time you enter a training program in surgery until you exit it five to seven years later, you are repeatedly called on to defend your actions and your decisions. At the staff level it is no different. All complications must be acknowledged and individual responsibility admitted. Surgeons play a game of one-upmanship on a daily basis. They hate to be wrong. The sense of competition is omnipresent.

In those days, our daily meetings were well attended. Today there are no regular meetings on a day-to-day basis; but back then, irrespective of the patient's clinical condition, we were there. On this day, Monica's third day post-surgery, the room was filled to overflowing. There were many possibilities raised, and unanimity seemed impossible. It was clear, however, that we were headed for a disaster unless an accurate diagnosis would permit specific and effective therapy to be initiated.

In retrospect, the lack of unanimity saved Monica's life. Had we agreed on a diagnosis and a course of action, she would likely not have survived. As it turned out, the correct diagnosis was never entertained that evening. The disparity of opinion led to the suggestion that the incision be opened, the lung inspected, and a biopsy of the lung taken. The decision to undertake this, given her condition, was a brave one. Concern was expressed that the operation itself would lead to further lung damage. That was a legitimate source of anxiety and there was certainly not a lot of room for error. Nonetheless, our failure to agree indicated that there was little choice in the matter. We at least had to have some idea of the problem if we were going to be able to reverse the downward spiral. The decision was by no means unanimous, but Joel, Alex, and I clearly were of the same opinion.

Thus the operation went ahead. To our delight there were no problems. Indeed, early lung biopsy would become a fairly routine part of our practice for the first few years of the program, to be replaced in later years by both experience and improved technology. The answer was swift. Toronto General Hospital is blessed with talented pathologists, not the least of which is a fellow named Dean Chamberlain (appropriately named, for he would soon become the "Dean" of Canadian pulmonary pathologists). The diagnosis was an entity known as diffuse alveolar damage—an alveolus is the medical term for the air sac where oxygen and carbon dioxide are exchanged. The diagnosis is also referred to as respiratory distress syndrome (RDS). I note its other name as a means of explaining the cause of the condition. Basically it isn't known.

Whenever you see the word "syndrome" appear, it is a hint that the cause of the problem remains obscure and all that the physicians know is that there is a grouping of clinical signs and symptoms associated with a particular pathological group of observations. It all sounds erudite, but basically, despite the accurate description, the physicians know very little in terms of causation or—as docs like to say—etiology. That is not to say that there hasn't been a great deal of effort expended to describe and validate the observations and establish the associated relevancies. Yet it sometimes takes several generations to establish cause and effect. In that regard, most of the infectious diseases that are of commonplace knowledge to school children today were very accurately described for hundreds of years before someone recognized that there was such a thing as a micro-organism. Back then they were called syndromes, plaques, or fevers. Although the description of the disease process might have been accurate, recognition of the cause or "etiology" awaited another generation.

Thus in 1984 not only were we still uncertain as to what had caused this pathological picture, there was controversy over its treatment. For a short time prior to 1984, intensive care physicians were convinced that the use of short-term high-dose steroid medication (cortisone) would be effective in treating the RDS. Although there was still some support for this therapy, most of us were beginning to recognize that such therapy was probably more deleterious in the long run. The popularity of cortisone was waning in the treatment of RDS. Consequently, when we came to discuss the initiation of steroids in Monica, there was little initial enthusiasm. As a result, there was a group of us who raised the possibility of adding cortisone to the armamentarium of therapy already in force.

Cortisone, or steroids, you will remember are also an anti-rejection drug, but one that we were avoiding in the early post-operative period because of Joel Cooper and Oriani Lima's work on the healing of the bronchial suture line alluded to in chapter two. In fact, we were convinced at that time that the avoidance of steroids had been responsible for our first success with Tom Hall. The major difference between the steroid therapy of RDS and of rejection is the length of therapy. As prophylaxis against rejection, steroids are a daily medication, whereas only a few doses were recommended for the therapy of RDS.

Surgeons are interventionalists, sometimes to the detriment of their patients, but often to their benefit. They are perturbed by inaction. Letting nature take its course and waiting for an accurate infallible diagnosis to initiate therapy is anathema. As surgeons directed every facet of the program in those early days, it is not therefore surprising that the decision was to treat Monica with steroids, sensing that if this was rejection, her condition had a reasonable chance of responding. There seemed little else we could offer, and such action certainly satisfied our anxiety more than did procrastination.

Monica began to improve two days later, and the process of healing accelerated thereafter. Her new lung showed signs of enhanced gas exchange before the chest x-ray reluctantly provided us with the realization that this improvement in oxygenation was not just more efficient delivery via the ventilator but was actually due to the recovery of the lung itself. In fact, she recovered faster than Tom Hall and was released from hospital with no requirement for a return to the intensive care unit.

Today we know that the diagnosis was respiratory distress syndrome, likely on the basis of inadequate lung preservation. We would soon change our procedures for ensuring that the donor lung did not deteriorate following extraction and while waiting for implantation. The other piece of the puzzle was not known in 1984. We knew at that time that RDS might not be improved by a short course of steroids. However, a decade later it was discovered that when given over a longer period of time (as we did here), steroids are effective in the treatment of RDS from whatever cause. As it turns out, we gave the correct treatment for the wrong reasons.

Such are the vagaries of medicine. Indeed, history may change the interpretation that I have put on this today, for we still don't know all the causes of RDS. Nonetheless, it is my presumption that the RDS was due to inadequate preservation and that steroids provided the answer. This is also the difference between the art and the science of medicine. Science is great, but only when you have all the answers. When the answers elude you, one needs the art, which, as in Monica's case, might prove advantageous even if for the wrong reasons.

The discrepancy in the size of her two lungs was dramatic to witness on an x-ray. Before and after transplant, chest x-rays illustrated that the new left lung occupied so much of her small body that one might wonder how Monica could avoid tilting to the left side. This is despite the fact that Bob Ginsberg had actually removed some of the transplanted lung in order to facilitate the closure of the chest. Joel Cooper was none the wiser about that slight addition to her operation until two years later when the matter of Monica's operation was raised at one of our transplant symposia.

During a panel discussion, Joel, as the chairman of the panel, was informing this international audience as to how we had come to the decision to use the left lung. During the discussion he did give me the credit for the suggestion to employ the left lung, a suggestion that two years later seemed so simple as to make me wish for anonymity on that score. Bob, while sitting on the same panel, quickly pointed out that while the selection of the left side had been important, the removal of a portion of the donor lung had also contributed to the accurate matching of the lung to the interior of the chest cavity. When Joel objected and noted that we had actually decided not to remove a portion of lung, Bob walked up to the radiology view box and drew his attention to a difficult-to-see row of stainless steel staples that cut a swath across the apex of Monica's new lung. Although surgeons' egos must find an outlet, and one might argue that this was not the ideal place or time to expose our duplicity, it did draw an amused ripple of comment from the audience.

Thus, at the end of 1984, there were two survivors of the single lung transplant procedure. As surgeons like to say—when you have done one case, you say "in my experience." When you have done two cases, you can say "in my series." And when you have done three, you are permitted to say "we see this over and over and over again." We had a series by this definition, and Tom's operation was no longer regarded as an exception to the rule. The two of them were wonderful examples of what sheer grit and determination in medicine could provide—to all of us they became known as the Dynamic Duo whenever they appeared in public on our behalf. A picture from one such event (Figure 10) shows Tom in the centre surrounded by Monica on his right and Ann Harrison, the world's first double lung recipient (more about her later), on his left.

As a result, a third single lung would quickly follow—a banker from Florida. With this notoriety came acceptance by the medical community, as three successes in a row could not be labelled coincidence. More important, however, was the confidence created within the community of patients. Applications to the program mushroomed, especially from the United States. In fact, for the next few years the majority of our patients were to be Americans, including the third single lung recipient, the bank manager from Florida.

The transplant symposia were to begin the following year as we related our experience and knowledge to the rest of the thoracic surgical world. It was a heady time for all of us. But as the program expanded and the number of potential recipients

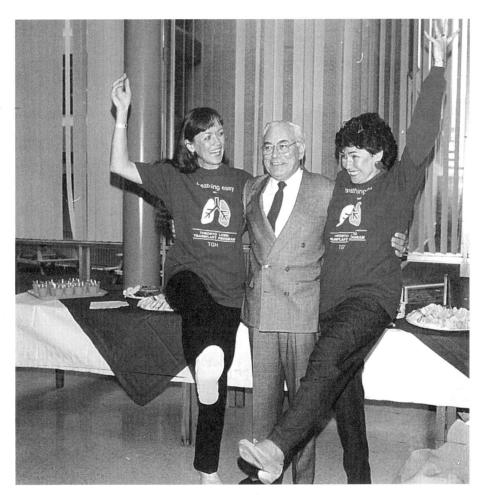
**Figure 10. Monica, Tom, and Ann Harrison
(the world's first double lung recipient) at a transplant fundraiser.**

grew, we were faced for the first time with the Achilles heel of transplantation: insufficient donors to meet the demand. It was difficult and depressing to lose a patient in the post-transplant period to complications or rejection. It was agonizing, however, to have a patient die on the waiting list from their underlying disease, waiting for the salvation that could have come but didn't. The problem with donors would become the next hurdle.

CHAPTER 7

The problem with donors
A death for a life

The problem with donors extends far beyond the fact that they are the rate-limiting step for solid organ transplantation. There are many issues that affect both the availability and selection of donors. These involve both physicians and the public. Issues of ethics, the definition of brain death, and legal and religious principles, all come together to create an aura of emotion and distress that is felt by all members of the medical team. The liver, kidney, heart, and lungs require an intact blood supply at the time of extraction as opposed to a corneal or bone transplant, which can be taken after the heart has stopped functioning. The heart must continue to pump oxygenated blood right up to the point where the organ is extracted or at least until a surgeon can insert a catheter into the artery supplying that organ to initiate the infusion of a preservative solution. Thus, the transplantation of these organs is only possible when "brain death" has occurred and the cardiovascular system continues to function normally. Once the traditional definition of death has occurred (i.e. the heart has stopped), damage to these organs is so rapid that transplantation is impossible.

Living-related donation was, until recently, only possible in the case of kidney transplantation simply because there were two organs and also because the donor operation is low risk. It has, however, become possible to remove part of the liver and transplant this portion into the appropriate recipient. This has been undertaken successfully from parent to child wherein the portion removed is quite sufficient to sustain the child. In addition, the liver is capable of rather phenomenal regeneration in both the recipient and the donor, and after several years it is apparent that the donor liver is growing in the child. In addition, the donor's remaining liver also appears to grow in size, as evidenced on CT scanning.

Despite such innovations, the removal of a portion of the liver is a much more serious undertaking than the extraction of one of the kidneys. The complication and indeed the mortality rate are higher, making it unlikely that this operative technique will be extended to unrelated recipients. It is one thing for a parent to accept such a risk for the life of his or her child, but quite another for a stranger or even a distantly related individual.

Of importance to a thoracic surgeon, donation from a living relative has also taken place in the field of lung transplantation wherein a *single lobe* has been provided from parent to child. There are reported cases of a lobe donated from each of the parents so that there is sufficient pulmonary volume to sustain the child. Once again, the risks of removal of a portion of your lung are substantially higher than for removal of the kidney. Removal of a whole lung, which would be a prerequisite for transplantation to another adult, carries an operative mortality of approximately five percent. That is, five of every 100 procedures will result in the death of the patient. With time, perhaps by the time this book hits the bookshops, this will occur with decreasing frequency.

Thus, "living-related donation" has little impact on the donor shortage. As a result, the clinical scenarios that permit solid organ donation are restricted to those cases where there has been sufficient brain damage from whatever event as to render the now potential donor incapable of sustained life. We refer to this as "brain death." The definition of brain death or the diagnosis of the condition varies amongst jurisdictions. Although this may at times create medical legal problems, in essence each definition describes a neurological condition for which the prognosis is hopeless and indeed the cessation of all bodily functions occurs within several hours or days of the diagnosis being rendered. If this were not the case, the surgical procedures that remove the vital organs of such individuals could be construed as the mechanism whereby their life was terminated, for other than irreversible neurological damage, the body is functioning normally. Therefore, the physicians must be satisfied that the extent of neurological damage warrants discontinuance of life support even if transplantation were not considered an option. In other words, the patient either serves as a donor or life support systems are withdrawn.

Many ICU physicians, such as myself, are involved in transplant programs. To avoid conflicts of interest, most transplant hospitals proscribe such physicians from declaring brain death if their particular organ of interest might be transplanted. Indeed, most hospitals have in place policies and procedures for the declaration of brain death. The institutional policies on brain death are sufficiently restrictive that they are more likely to result in patients' being maintained in a vegetative state for some time—or the loss of donor organs—than the inappropriate declaration of brain death. The donor is frequently lost because of a rapid progression of cerebral and pulmonary dysfunction resulting in the demise of the patient before the donation process could be fully completed. That is the price exacted for the assurance of accuracy.

Despite this practice, in the early 1980s there was no uniform rule for the declaration of brain death between hospitals and jurisdictions. At times, this led to embarrassing problems for the health care system. Witness the problem that I noted in Chapter 3. I had transported a donor back from Atlanta, Georgia, totally relying on the neurological assessment done in Georgia as indicative that brain death had occurred. However, once in Canada, the diagnosis could not be made according to our criteria.

I remember another situation that occurred within the confines of Toronto. A potential donor had been identified at St. Michael's hospital, another of the teaching institutions at the University of Toronto. The facility is a mere ten-minute car ride from Toronto General. The patient in question had been declared brain dead by two physicians at St Michael's, one of whom was the University Professor and head of Neurosurgery. Given this declaration and the fact that the family had provided consent for all organs, the ophthalmologists there had proceeded to remove the eyes for corneal grafts. Corneal grafts are utilized at the individual hospital, and there is no sharing mechanism between hospitals. Thus they fall outside the normal mechanism of donation, and usually donation takes place at the hospital where declaration has occurred. St Michael's, however, would not permit us operating room time for the other organs, and therefore the patient was transferred to Toronto General. Such refusals were commonplace in the late 1980s as individual hospitals within the province of Ontario tried to protect their budgets.

Unfortunately, the patient arrived at the General hypothermic. To be declared brain dead at our institution, the body temperature must be at or near normal. Thus, we could not declare brain death. This of course provided for no small amount of concern and embarrassment, as the declaration had been performed by the university's most respected neurosurgeon; and of course the eyes had already been removed. The scenario presented a rather untidy public relations problem. How do you explain to the family of the donor all the delays before the body could be released? With some verbal dexterity, one could perhaps explain the fact that donor criteria varied between institutions. However, I would not want to be the one to handle the queries as to why the eyes were removed if the patient was not brain dead by the Toronto General standards. No matter how logical the explanation and notation of the fact that brain death according to our standards was inevitable, the mere mention of variable criteria for organ donation would send any member of the family into a fit of understandable outrage. I really don't know how the public relations aspect was solved, but fortunately the donor/patient did eventually meet our criteria as expected.

In summary, then, most solid organ transplant donation must occur from a brain-dead individual in whom the organ function appears normal by all standard testing. Consequently, a tragedy must provide the second chance at life for the anxiously waiting recipient. A sudden or accidental death is the prerequisite for the subsequent transplant to occur—in other words, a death for a life. The organs of young persons are preferable, and the commonest cause of death under the age of forty is trauma or a sudden cerebral hemorrhage. In this regard, the transplantation process has all the required elements of any theatrical tragedy. The medical team steps onto a roller coaster ride of emotion each time it receives a call that a donor has been found. It is just very difficult to handle a situation that is tragic and aesthetically unpleasant but which at the same time provides unimaginable joy for the recipient and their families.

The donor organizations euphemistically refer to the donation process as an opportunity for new life to begin as if that somehow mitigates the despair and anguish of those who have lost their loved one suddenly under tragic circumstances. It is referred to as a "new start" for a stranger who would have perished were it not for the unwitting gift of life from another person now referred to as "the donor." All that is true.

You might ask why the process is aesthetically unpleasant for the medical team. Picture this reality. The surgeon on the donor team arrives in the operating room to safely extract the organs for the intended recipient. Unlike in his/her normal practice, the patient is an unknown entity other than for the information that the transplant coordinator has provided. You know the age—they are usually young. You are aware of the circumstances that have brought them to this unfortunate end—a car accident, a spontaneous brain hemorrhage, a cardiac arrest that has resulted in successful cardiovascular resuscitation but has left them "brain dead." You are also aware of their vital signs, fully knowledgeable of the fact that there is a blood pressure, that the organs you are here to extract are functional. At times you may be told that the situation is precarious—that the blood pressure is already unstable, that the oxygenation is declining rapidly, that there is some urgency to proceed to extraction before a full-blown cardiac arrest occurs or before irreversible damage to "your" organ occurs.

But you know little of the patients themselves. Occasionally you are aware of the social history that may be relevant to what you are about to do. On other occasions the sheer scope of the tragedy is related to you simply because of its perceived magnitude. I recall one instance where I arrived in the operating room in another provincial capital to be informed that this sixteen-year-old donor had been struck from behind by a drunk driver while riding his bike home from school. He was the only son of one of the local surgeons. The anaesthetist on duty that night knew the family well. There was a stillness in the room that was palpable and the demeanour of the anaesthetist cast a shadow over us all.

There was another case in the United states where the young woman upon whom I was about to operate was the second daughter and only surviving child of a woman who had lost her husband and her older daughter to a motor vehicle accident only two years previously. The beginning of a new life for some unknown patient in a faraway city was little compensation for the tragedy experienced by this unfortunate parent. It is this reality that is presented to the donor team.

Most of the time, donor operations take place in the stillness of the after-hour shifts and usually in other cities and unfamiliar hospitals. It all occurs following a cold and uncomfortable trip during hours when you would normally be asleep. The corridors of the hospital are quiet and the operating rooms and lounges empty but for somebody's half-eaten supper on a table, some scattered newspapers, and the ubiquitous blanket and pillow discarded with abandon on a couch; all signs of an anaesthetist and nurses on shift. There is no glory here; no sense of excitement. The OR nurses are frequently subdued and reserved. It is apparent that on some occasions it is because they feel the surgeons from the tertiary care centre will be demanding or require a level of expertise on their part that they are incapable of fulfilling. Mostly, however, it is related to a distaste for the event that is about to take place.

The atmosphere in the recipient operating room at Toronto General provides a stark contrast. The place hums. Everyone is delighted to be there anticipating the excitement and drama that accompanies a lung transplant. The patient will be euphoric coming into the room. Nurses are chattering at each other over instruments, and coordinators are constantly asking you for details on the case. What instruments do you need for this one? Are we likely to go on bypass? Do you want the pump in the room? Where is the donor from? Do you want blood in the room? Are we doing a double? It goes on. There are always physician visitors lounging about, surgeons or trainees who have been staying in Toronto waiting to see what is about to unfold. Their enthusiasm permits you to relive the underlying excitement you felt with the first one, and their sense of participating in a unique surgical experience is infectious. They follow you everywhere, anxious to learn. The ones who cannot converse well in English are a bit of a challenge. They tend not to understand that you are actually just walking down the corridor to the washroom and not to the operating theatre to commence the procedure. You can sense their awkwardness as they follow you to the urinal.

In the donor room, you don't have visiting physicians and surgeons craning their necks over the drapes or standing on stools to observe your every move. It's the middle of the night in a distant city. There are no visitors here, other than you. Everyone who doesn't have to be there is at home and fast asleep. Here in the donor room, despite the fact that the operation is just as complex and just as subject to intra-operative catastrophes, the atmosphere is somber. There is no sense of adventure. Everyone here knows that at the end of the procedure there will not be a patient who has been provided with a new lease on life. There will be no relieved and grateful family members attendant on your every word in the waiting room. Rather, there is a body that was once a human being special to people that you know are grieving quietly elsewhere. Rather than a return to the excitement of the ICU with a fresh recipient, there is a covered gurney that is quietly pushed down the hall to the pathology department. At least I get to travel back to Toronto and witness first hand the positive side of the process. For the donor hospital staff, it is simply as described.

As a result, upon arrival in a strange operating room I usually attempt to be, if not euphoric, then at least outgoing and upbeat in my attitude. Frequently a few words about the recipient back in Toronto, some details of who he is, the anguish of his disease, and the incredible impact that a successful donor operation will have on his life helps provide some relief from the all-too-apparent tragedy of the patient who lies on the table. The donor's status is in full view, whereas that of the recipient is unknown to the donor hospital team. It has always seemed appropriate to provide the recipient information to these folks who are a long way from the excitement of the transplant itself.

It is hard not to refer to the patient as a patient while I write this, but indeed in reality we always referred to the person on the table as the "donor." Perhaps that is part of the desensitization process that medical folks must develop. Nonetheless, it is also hard to regard him or her as a patient when you are fully aware that your operation, despite being skillfully done, will result in their demise. Sure, he/she is brain dead—all that is true. But in the end, the cessation of all other bodily functions will be at your instigation; it will be created by your hands.

This is particularly true for the cardiac and thoracic teams. Although the liver team normally proceeds first as far as dissection of the organs is concerned, it is the cardiac and thoracic surgeons who commence the withdrawal of the organs themselves. It is they who create the circumstance that causes the heart to cease its function and the circulation to stop. The liver team does a detailed and complex dissection of all the vital structures required for the eventual removal of the liver. Then the cardiac and/or thoracic surgeon performs a dissection of the major blood vessels entering and exiting the heart and lungs. These latter operators also insert cannulas or catheters in the aorta and into the pulmonary artery to enable their assistants to commence the infusion of a cold electrolyte solution containing chemicals designed to protect the organ during the time it is without its circulation. This is the "preservation" we have spoken of before.

The dissections are as technically demanding, if not more so, than any other thoracic procedure. An error could result in the loss of not just the organ you came to "harvest," but in the failure of the other surgical teams to obtain their organs as well, hence affecting several different recipients in diverse cities throughout North America. That your technical error could result in the death of the patient/donor should seem unimportant, as the subject of all your operative skills is already brain dead. Yet an error here could result in the death of more than one individual; the mortality rates on the recipient waiting list are as high as twenty-five to thirty percent.

At least that is what you steel your mind to as you stand there waiting for the OR staff to be ready. The cannulas are in place and in your hand you hold a syringe. The syringe contains a substance called PGE1 or prostaglandin E1. Injected into the main pulmonary artery, it will dilate the vessels to permit an even distribution of the cold preservative mixture throughout the lung without a concomitant rise in the pressure within the pulmonary vessels that might be damaging to the lung. It also will cause the other vessels in the body to dilate and the blood pressure will begin to fall. In other words, the substance produces a shock-like state. I usually watch the pressure falling on the monitor over the drapes. We all do.

As the systolic blood pressure reaches about fifty millimetres of mercury, we tie off the superior vena cava, the main source of blood return to the heart from the upper part of the body. At this point, the heart usually arrests and the various infusion solutions, ice-cold from the coolers we have brought with us, are commenced. There is a great deal more of surgical detail, but in essence it is now over for the donor/patient. The heart has now stopped and clinical death as lay people know it has occurred; right there in the operating room and under my hand and supervision. The anaesthetist turns off the ventilator. His/her part is now over.

Once the infusion is done, either I or a heart surgeon, if the heart is to be used, remove the heart followed by both lungs still attached to the trachea. When it is all finished, the chest cavity is empty save for the esophagus snaking its way to the stomach below the diaphragm. The only other time I have seen an empty body cavity was in the autopsy suite. There it is normal, but here in the operating room, at the conclusion of a successful surgery, it is an eerie sight. I like to be gone as quickly as possible.

That's why it is aesthetically unpleasant. A surgeon operates to save a life. Like other physicians, that is the *raison d'être* of your craft. Here you must end a life in order to provide a chance at life for your recipient who waits in another operating room in another city with another team of surgeons. You would prefer to be on the latter team. You recognize the fact that brain death has occurred and that you are not the one to really end this life (although that has been contested in criminal cases when the donor's injury is the result of an assault). Yet, you are left with the sense that you ravaged this patient and at times (especially when not in your own hospital) you think about the declaration of brain death. You didn't do it yourself. You don't even know the ones who undertook the examination and you are definitely unaware as to whether there might be confounding variables that would have affected the ultimate decision.

When I first started as director of the donor program, I insisted that the donor still be in the intensive care unit when I arrived. I wanted—actually needed—to do the examination myself. I wanted to assure myself that this patient/donor was truly brain dead by my criteria and those of my own hospital. That certainly prolonged the time I was away on the donor run. It also began to hold up the other donor teams, and it wasn't long before I was no longer able to undertake this piece of personal reassurance. Now all the preparation is done locally and the patient/donor is already in the operating room and fully draped for surgery when we arrive. Only the head is visible, and that is behind the screen that separates the surgeon and anaesthetist. The depersonalization is complete. In fact, unless the lungs are the only organs to be utilized, the liver team has already started the operation. As a result, you don't know much about the donor. Perhaps that is best.

The consent process itself poses an ethical and logistical dilemma for the ICU physician. As the physician in charge of maintaining the potential donor, one must be wary of addressing the possibilities of organ donation unless you are certain that brain death has supervened. Thus before the reality of brain death itself is at hand, the family has had no time to reflect on the principles of organ donation, let alone the reality of actually assenting to the use of the organs from their loved one. Therefore, it is usually not until after the announcement of brain death that the family is approached about organ donation.

Occasionally, a family aware of the neurological assessment underway and its possible consequences will initiate the discussion. If that occurs, it makes the entire process more comfortable, but even then it is not an easy interaction for anyone. It always bothered me in my capacity as an intensive care doctor to have to provide the devastating news that the situation was indeed hopeless and then follow that with the request to obtain the organs of the brain-dead, but not yet officially deceased, loved one of the family sitting across from me. The timing could not be more awkward. Yet, once the pronouncement of death is made, the next of kin may no longer be accessible, and thus the request is usually made at this time of heightened emotion and distress.

It is all a matter of judgment and timing. I have always attempted to have another member of the team with me—a nurse or pastoral care advisor—and the two of us assess each situation for the optimal timing of our request. Nonetheless, it remains an uncomfortable moment. The grief reaction is variable, and it is important to observe the family members carefully before proclaiming the verdict.

I was always concerned to ascertain, as early as possible, the dynamics of the family. Hopefully you have had a chance to speak with them previously. This affords you the opportunity to assess their composure, to determine who are the leaders, and the ones most likely to hear as well as listen. Are you going to need a pastoral care worker or social worker or both present when you confirm their worst fears?

This is such an important aspect of delivering bad news that many physicians will indicate at the initial interaction that things are grim and the prognosis is not optimistic even when it is already obvious that brain death is inevitable or already present. Such provides some time for the family to adjust before the final verdict. The fact that the ultimate declaration requires the assessment of two physicians often affords the opportunity to begin to develop a relationship with the family and at least form an initial impression of the family dynamics. Frequently, however, one is overwhelmed with the work in the unit, and the assessment of the family is compressed into a few anxious moments. Commonly, important family members are delayed in their arrival, necessitating delivering the tragic news with no preparation.

It is never easy; but always it is most difficult when the penultimate meeting is also the first. Faced with that circumstance, it was my practice to prepare the way as best I could by initially explaining the circumstances, outlining what had happened, and what we had attempted to do. With each piece of the puzzle that you give them, the inevitability of what is about to come becomes more and more obvious. As this happens, you can see understanding appear in the eyes of some while in others even the final pronouncement remains unheard and obscure. Even after you have said words such as "The situation is not recoverable," "He cannot recover from this," "There is no hope," or the often-phrased, "It is just a matter of time," incomprehension persists. They look wide-eyed about the room with tears welling in their eyes and say, "But he is going to recover, isn't he?" It is only when you affirmatively say NO to that question that reality dawns. Those are the situations that distress me the most. That is when I find asking for organ donation, not in the next breath, but during that same interaction, repulsive, if not impossible. I have lost donors by offering my sympathies, excusing myself and leaving them in the hands of the others, intending to return. But sometimes you don't have an opportunity to return, or the immediate next of kin leaves before you get a second chance. Sometimes you just can't bring yourself to ask even on the second attempt. Their grief can be so overwhelming, so heartfelt, and sometimes so violently expressive—pounding their fists on the wall, screaming their dismay, and sometimes accusing you of ineptitude— that the mere query appears overly intrusive.

On such occasions, donors are lost. Unfortunately, there is an even greater number of potential donors who were never considered for the donation process. The reasons for this loss are legion. Physicians forget. In other circumstances the physician is ignorant of the fact that this brain-dead individual might be an organ donor. Most doctors are unaware of the specific requirements for each donor organ—not surprising, as the prerequisites may change annually, and the requirements for organ donation are not likely to find their way into publications read by the average physician. Hyper-specialization has seen to it that medical publications are segregated into specialty journals.

For example, our early requirements for lung donation included an age under fifty years, non-smoking status, a clear chest x-ray, and oxygen levels in the arterial blood greater than 300 millimetres of mercury. Most physicians, coordinators, and other paramedical staff regarded these criteria as sacrosanct, the result of intensive research and/or experience. In reality, they were the result of an early Sunday morning impromptu coffee session between Joel Cooper and myself. Joel asked me what criteria I thought would constitute the ideal donor. After some thought and another cup of coffee, we came up with the criteria noted above. It is important to remember that we determined all this in the early days when we were just beginning the program and were anxious to ensure its success.

Thus every attempt was made to provide for the ideal circumstance. Approximately ten years later, I was attending a major thoracic surgical convention and was in the audience when a surgical training resident from an American University presented a paper that in essence attempted to expand the criteria for the lung donor. During the discussion a senior surgeon from the American south castigated the young presenter, and was highly critical of such efforts to liberalize the donor criteria. He was concerned that such would endanger the good results currently being experienced throughout North America. I had no objection to a call for a caution but when he pompously proclaimed that the current criteria were tried and true having been accurately worked out in the early days of lung transplantation, I was aghast. The poor surgeon on the podium looked abashed and embarrassed, and I found myself at the microphone explaining to the assembly the true origin of the "tried and true" criteria.

Unfortunately, we sometimes accept the casual as the credible. Indeed, by 1989 we were accepting donors between fifty and sixty years of age. A history of smoking was permitted if all else looked reasonable. An abnormal chest x-ray became permissible if it was just in the one lung and oxygenation was satisfactory. Time holds nothing constant. If the thoracic surgeons seemed unclear as to the donor criteria for lungs, one could hardly expect emergency room and ICU physicians to be more cognizant of the requirements. The message of the donor acquisition agencies remains: *ask the family every time!* Consider every brain-dead individual a potential donor. Until physicians adopt that mindset, organ donation will continue to be a fraction of the possible. Potential recipients on transplant waiting lists will continue to succumb of their disease processes unless the donor pool expands.

The interminable wait for a donor is mirrored on the faces of the recipients as they sit around the conference room before their weekly support session commences. The sessions are chaired by social service or the recipient coordinator, but frequently one of the medical team is invited to attend; I was afforded several opportunities to observe their sessions. The patients and their support persons are all in attendance. Some walk into the room pulling their oxygen tanks; others require wheelchairs. They may be so young as to break your heart with their youthfulness gone wrong. Others are older and quiet. But they are all old in spirit. The support persons assist them but seem even more anxious for the meeting to commence. They wait to hear how their colleagues are faring after transplantation and, more important, to learn why one of their number is *not* in attendance. The questions are asked discreetly—"Is he sick?" "How are we doing for donors?"

I attended one such meeting at a time when a donor drought was prolonged and just after we had launched the distant retrieval aspect of the program. I knew that they were excited about the possibility of our obtaining additional donors by travelling to other centres to perform the donor operation.

Ostensibly I was there to provide hope that this new approach would quickly bring to each of them their long-sought salvation. It had been several weeks without a transplant. Amongst the very fragile ones you can readily see the strain, the worry etched on faces that are one moment drawn and weary and the next forcing a smile and a laugh at the quip you make from the front of the room in an effort to provide encouragement.

But they have waited six to eighteen months, and for some the predicted length of their possible survival has come and gone. They have been admitted to hospital with increasing frequency and recognize that soon we will inform them that they are too ill to continue on the program. Eventually they are admitted to hospital full time and arrive at the support group meeting in a wheelchair on high-flow oxygen. There is a strained silence that comes over the group when they are recognized by the chairperson to address the assembly. All in attendance are fully aware of their status and that this could be their last session. I have heard them ask if there are new ideas for the acquisition of donors; if we have been able to broaden our area of acquisition.

On one such occasion a young woman virtually apologized for addressing the issue, "I'm sorry to press," she said, "but as you can see, I don't have a lot of time to wait for this to happen."

They also are aware that as deterioration progresses, the chances they will survive the procedure begins to decrease. At that time the program was still a fledgling and any sudden increase in mortality rates would have seen the hospital end all our activity. In fact, the insurers for the US patients still refused to remunerate us in the late 1980s, stating that we provided an experimental treatment. We all were performing a balancing act. Everyone understood the rules of the game. We were in business to bring folks back from the brink of impending death but the closer they came to the edge, the more their systems became impaired, the more likely we would repudiate the contract we had made with them. We were simply trying to reduce risk, minimize bad outcomes, and thereby preserve the program. As the years wore on, we would become more aggressive but there would always be that challenge to maintain excellent results. There would always be a group of professionals in the program who were conservative in their approach. Those looked strictly at outcomes and statistics. If they had had the reins at the outset of the program we would never have performed the first transplant.

We always tried to terminate the patient sessions with some good news, providing information on the successful patients who had left hospital and were now back home. Frequently, Tom Hall or Monica Assenheimer would attend and provide a real-life testimony to the fact that hope did exist. There were also the quips that in any other forum might sound callous but were designed to provide a degree of black humour to relieve the tension of the moment. If a long weekend were approaching, I've heard it said to the gathering, "Best be sure your pagers are working—business will be good!" I've also had the patients suggest that I should check out the age and size of pedestrians before running the orange light or perhaps even the red one. "Surely the cops would understand!" they would laugh.

None of our potential recipients actually wished the death of another, but that is not to say they didn't pray that if and when an accidental death occurred the victim might at least have their blood type and approximate them in chest dimensions. For they all know that there will be accidental deaths day after day, year by year. The problem is converting the traumatic fatality into a donor. The latter occurs rarely, and perhaps there lies the real tragedy in this era of expanded transplant capability.

At the end of one such session, I was approached by the mother of a patient with cystic fibrosis. Her daughter of twenty years was deteriorating rapidly and we had not performed a transplant in six weeks. Although this was distinctly better than the early days when transplants occurred every six months, it was by this time considered a drought.

"Has anyone been transplanting lungs these past few weeks?" she asked. The real question was in her eyes: *Are you guys just not accepting the donors because you want perfection?* And she followed with the essence of the matter for her: "Would you be willing to relax the donor criteria for her? I know you can't say you will, but please think about it if one comes through for her."

I wanted to reassure her that we would definitely find that elusive donor for her daughter. But that was not to be. The drought lasted for another two weeks and when they started to come again, it was too late for that young woman and her mother. They had waited in Toronto for over a year. The mother was left to clear out her belongings from their meagre apartment and leave the city to return home alone.

The scarcity of donors and the anxiety attendant upon their acquisition presents an ongoing problem for the transplant program staff that at times assumes an ethical dimension. Although this will be discussed further in subsequent chapters, an example here seems appropriate. Daniel was one of our early group of potential recipients that emigrated to Toronto after the successes of Tom and Monica. He was a great man. Wonderfully understanding of the entire process, he displayed a compassion for his peers that endeared him to everyone. Despite his own severe problems from pulmonary fibrosis, he had time for others in the program when time had little left for him. There was never an urgency to his actions or questions. He was relaxed and, like Tom Hall, accepting of his fate. He was concerned at the distress felt by his compatriots in the program and provided strength and support when indeed, from a medical point of view, he seemed to be the most fragile of all.

It thus seemed appropriate that he underwent a successful single lung transplant in the nick of time and enjoyed an unremarkable post-operative course. His compassion and caring for others within the program did not decrease following his own optimistic outcome. With each visit to the clinic for follow-up, each physiotherapy session, and all the support group sessions, which he faithfully attended, Daniel was an active participant in the reassurance of others. He calmed their concerns and apprehensions—a true rock in the storm. However, at six months, rejection became an unfortunate reality. Hospitalization and augmentation of his immunosuppression became necessary. Though improved temporarily, he would never return to the immediate post-transplant state. Multiple admissions for either further episodes of rejection or for infection secondary to the increased immunosuppression ensued. His confidence never failed him in public and his grit in the face of continued adversity provided inspiration for others.

There did come a time when oxygen dependence returned despite all efforts to manage his problems. The recurrent trauma to the new lung wrought by rejection and infection simply proved too much and permanent scarring was obviously present on his x-ray.

One evening, Daniel and I were able to speak quietly together. My day had finished, and there was a rare moment of uncommitted time. I was distressed with myself that I had seen him only briefly during his most recent admission. In the quiet of his room he indicated to me that he realized that there was no further hope for him, no chance to reverse the changes brought by the rejection of what had seemed initially to be a great success. He asked what options lay ahead, though he knew them as well as I did. There does come a time, however, when a patient really has to ask the obvious; a time when he or she will seek bold, uncompromising confirmation by the physician. I considered carefully my answer; and I suppose because Daniel opened the Pandora's Box, I asked him whether he would consider undergoing a second transplant procedure were it to be offered to him. There was no hesitation in his affirmative response.

With most patients, I would not have mentioned that option, simply because it had not been developed as policy within the program itself. Nonetheless, the program at that point in its history remained innovative, with a genuine desire to provide the "cutting edge" in pulmonary transplantation. I quickly told him that I was not speaking for the program. I anticipated that this entire question could unleash a wave of political pressure from various interest groups, both within and without the lung transplant program (physicians, psychologists, nurses, potential and transplanted recipients and their families).

But Daniel was to my mind different. He understood that I was speaking as his friend and as his advisor. In the program at that time, we felt that we owed the patients a thorough explanation of everything that might—just might—be possible. From that evening onward, I began to lobby to have Daniel accepted back onto the list for transplantation. In several quarters it was not a welcome suggestion because there were indeed legitimate issues that had to be addressed. Questions posed by members of the team (the size of which was increasing every month) included:

- Could we prove that his lung was irreparably damaged?

- If we did do a second transplant, should we transplant the other side; or remove the rejected lung and perform the second transplant on the same side?

- What priority should he be given on the waiting list?

This latter was the major question. First, it was suggested that he had had his chance and the provision of another lung might deprive another potential recipient of any chance at all. Second, it was questioned whether the risk of a second transplant was so high that it was unwarranted to waste the donor lung when it could be employed for a first-time recipient, raising a significant ethical dilemma to be discussed in depth later.

The entire matter was the subject of debate in open conversation and also behind closed doors amongst the leaders of the program. We were concerned as to the opinion of the others waiting on the list. Would they resent the fact that one of their number was to be given a second chance, perhaps at the expense of themselves? At that time, re-transplantation had yet to be undertaken, although it had occurred following heart/lung procedures and we had performed a second procedure on the other side for Jack Collins. The latter had occurred, however, before the program had acquired more than one recipient on the list.

The discussions concerning Daniel went on for some time.

Before a final decision could be reached, his time ran out. There was to be no second chance and our problem in ethical decision making could be deferred. Daniel and his family accepted our indecision and procrastination with equanimity. On only one occasion did I witness the steel of his resolution and acceptance of his fate waver. I spied him in a wheelchair at the elevator door about to head outdoors for some fresh air and to join the legions of employees and smokers who congregated on the back lawn on Elizabeth Street. After the usual pleasantries, he asked, "Any donors in sight for me?"

"None at all, Daniel—we're in a major drought," I answered.

Tears welled in those eyes that always held such mirth and his voice cracked ever so slightly as he said, "Well—you better hurry."

That was it. The elevator opened, and in a moment I was waving my last goodbye to a great gentleman. Sometimes, patients just seem to know when the end is at hand. When you are short of breath, it must seem like the end is always near; and the distress that Daniel felt that day must have been overwhelming. For Daniel, as for so many, the ordeal of waiting is too often punctuated by a decline in function and death before the salvation of the donor becomes a reality.

The fact of the matter is that there are too few donors. Despite their scarcity, there are many who feel that if everyone filled out their donor card, the problem would disappear. Yet the problem goes beyond donor consent. It is woven into the fabric of our consciousness, wherein we fail to acknowledge our own ultimate demise and have a profound inherent respect for those who have been touched by the unexpected loss of a loved one. The former affects the number of donor cards that are signed. A refusal to sign—we would not call it a refusal but a neglect—permits you to ignore the possibility that untimely death may occur. You aren't depriving anyone of a donor because you will not ever be in the position of being one—right? As far as the latter is concerned, physicians are culturally driven to provide support for the mourning family. As noted above, such frequently precludes posing the difficult question of organ donation to the family. Even when the family acknowledges the fact that the donor card was signed by their loved one, I have witnessed them pull back from sanctioning that expression of caring, by their inability to legally fulfill the consent process. Their pain is obvious. They know that their loved one wished to serve as an organ donor. Yet in the midst of their grief they cannot bear to consent to that final act upon the body of one they loved so much and grieve for so deeply.

Viewing the program from the recipient's perspective conditions the manner in which you approach donation and the process involved. Certainly the operative experience with the recipient, as noted, carries with it more hype and self-satisfaction. However, none of it can even begin to occur without the death of the donor and the orchestrated management of organ donation.

In an effort to maintain excellent outcomes, I have explained how the assessment of recipients had evolved to the selection of those best able to withstand the rigours of the operative and post-operative experience, while at the same time ensuring that their life expectancy was sufficiently limited to warrant the risks. The team was most anxious to acquire a donor for anyone on the recipient waiting list, given the twenty-five percent mortality that was consistent on an annual basis. As a result, there was considerable pressure to push the donor program to produce as many as possible.

However, those of us performing the donor selection tended to bring the same rigour to that process as the entire team did to the recipient selection. One wanted to produce the best results. If a donor lung performed badly immediately post-op, it was quickly concluded that the preservation, or the selection in the first place, had been faulty. In the early days, the balancing act was always onerous, especially as I continued to know the potential recipients well, participated fully in the recipient selection process, and directed the post-operative ICU care.

There were many occasions when I sat in my family room by the telephone in the dark hours of the night, struggling with the decision to proceed. The oxygen levels were lower than acceptable in the donor, or the chest x-ray was not quite normal (read by a non-radiologist physician whom I didn't know), or the donor was fifty-eight and a smoker. On the other hand, you can put a face on the problem. Based on blood type and size, you know who will be the potential recipient, a recipient who by this time has been notified to come as quickly as possible to the hospital. Rejecting the donor carries with it the sure knowledge that this may be the last chance for that recipient. Thus, donor rejection may imply recipient rejection as well.

The decision was even harder sitting in a foreign operating room lounge having travelled by aircraft for a few hours with one's team. Sometimes the decisions were straightforward. The oxygen levels had plummeted to a point where it would be madness to proceed. At other times the donor was doubtful but the recipient had been on the list for only a short period of time, was stable, and had a common blood type. There was a reasonable chance that another opportunity would arise for that individual. Yet, there were so many times when I fervently wished that the chest x-ray could be just a little more abnormal or the oxygen tensions somewhat lower—anything to make the decision more palatable and predictable.

On those occasions when I was sorely tempted to accept an unfavourable donor lung, I would remember the incidents when a less than ideal selection had proved fatal. I remember an unfortunate donor selection from our early days. It was shortly after the euphoria of Tom Hall and Monica Assenheimer. We were offered the lungs from a young drowning victim. As I write these words today, I find it difficult to believe that we actually accepted a drowning victim as a donor. Our recipient was in desperate straits. The donor had been out of the water for two days and the lungs were functioning beautifully. Not only was the chest x-ray pristine but the oxygen levels were the best we had ever seen.

My first reaction was to decline the offer because of the history of submersion, and I sorely wish I had paid heed to that warning in my head. But as the word spread through the program that there was such an excellent donor available, the pressure began for us to reconsider the decision. Thus, as the questions concerning my judgment increased, I found myself discussing the matter with Alec Patterson at the main desk in the ICU. As I noted, we were still bathing in our recent success and notoriety, and overconfidence is not unknown in surgeons. After reviewing the situation again and again, we decided to accept the donor and proceed with the transplant. Both Alec and I were confident.

The procedure went smoothly, but the recipient acquired a virulent pneumonia on the first post-operative day and died a few days later from progressive respiratory failure and sepsis. We had seen severe pneumonia in the past, but never so soon after surgery and rarely so aggressive and destructive. We became convinced that all this had occurred from our misjudgment in donor selection. As Joel would later remark when informed of the outcome and the circumstances leading up to it: "You did *what*? What were you guys thinking of?"

Since that incident I have observed the same virulent fatal pneumonia in other patients post-transplant, suggesting that it is possible that the sequence of events had nothing at all to do with the fact that the donor had been a drowning victim. However, having said that, I would not make the same decision again. Medicine is sometimes like that. Often our practice is dictated by our experience and the desire to avoid repeating supposed errors. Although this is a natural—and some would say appropriate and laudable—practice, it does mean that one bad outcome can preclude the acceptance of a practice that has basic merit. I doubt, however, if this one will ever be tested again.

Prior to 1986, I had had only one previous exposure to the donor operation. The circumstance had involved one of our early cases wherein the donor and the recipient operation were both performed in our hospital. While we were preparing the omentum in the recipient, an urgent call for assistance was made from the donor room. As Joel was the senior surgeon in the recipient room, he sent me down the hall. The problem was an inadvertent hole in one of the pulmonary veins. It wasn't a significant difficulty—all they required was some improved exposure to suture the vessel.

I wasn't there very long, but long enough to recognize the stark contrast in atmosphere between the two rooms. Thus when informed by Joel that the donor aspect of the program was to be my responsibility, I was less than pleased. As noted previously, my initial involvement in the donor program was as the director of the ICU. My assignment was to decrease the time between arrival of a donor in our ICU and the onset of the surgery. This was an organizational matter only and although I was not terribly pleased with the responsibility, I took it on without a great deal of thought as to what else it might portend.

Our success, however, had brought a steadily increasing number of recipients to the program, a number that would greatly exceed our ability to provide organs. We had at the outset insisted that the donors be brought to Toronto General. This afforded us the luxury of reducing the ischemic time of the transplanted lung. Ischemia is a medical term that refers to a condition of reduced oxygenated blood flow to an organ to the point where its function is potentially permanently impaired. The ischemic time refers to the time from the point of cessation of blood flow in the donor to the time it is re-established in the recipient. This is the time of greatest hazard to the transplanted lung. If all other factors are equal (and there are many other factors), then the overall function of the lung is inversely proportional to the ischemic time.

Unfortunately, however, a short ischemic time obtained from having donor and recipient in the same hospital greatly reduced the total number of available donors. There were two reasons for this. First, the families of the patient/donor were reluctant to grant permission to have their loved one flown to Toronto. Second, the time involved in the transfer of the patient increased the overall time from consent for donation to the actual surgery. It is a much more complex procedure to arrange air transport of the patient/donor than it is to send a surgical team to the hospital of origin. Once out of the ICU in an ambulance or aircraft, the donor is at greater risk of sustaining periods of unrecognized or inadequately treated low blood pressure. As I've noted elsewhere in these pages, the lung is an organ that deteriorates very quickly once brain death supervenes. It is also sensitive to changes in blood pressure. Reductions in blood pressure that are sufficiently severe as to result in a shock state are well known to lead to the development of pulmonary dysfunction due to the accumulation of water in the air sacs of the lung. Such can result in severe damage to the potential transplant even before the ischemic time has its onset.

Other transplant programs such as kidney, heart, and liver had for some time been retrieving their donor organs by transporting the surgical team to the hospital where the donor resided. At times, these teams would travel great distances to achieve their goal. As the number of programs increased through the late seventies and early eighties, it became commonplace for a variety of transplant teams from different centres to converge on the donor hospital at a pre-appointed time to commence the extraction of the organs. It was apparent that these programs were more mature and that they had developed unique means of preserving the organs during the ischemic period.

As noted above, preservation of these involved the intra-operative perfusion into the organ in question of a cold preservative solution that contained a variety of chemicals designed to reduce the damage done by protracted ischemia.

When it came to lung transplantation, it was clear that we were neophytes in the manner of donor acquisition. Our preservation of the lung consisted of collapsing the lungs after the arrest of the heart and then filling the thoracic cavity with ice-cold electrolyte solution. We had been so concerned with the recipient operation and his/her subsequent care that insufficient attention was paid to the first critical step in the process. However, without a viable donor lung, the recipient was unlikely to survive irrespective of surgical technique and post-operative skills.

Compared to the refinements of others, our technique seemed rather primitive. In retrospect, the only reason that we were able to manage with this technique was simply the fact that our ischemic times were short. The short ischemic time was the result of insisting that donors be brought to Toronto. It was rapidly becoming apparent that we had to conform to established practice if the program were to perform more than a few transplants annually. Clearly, the patients on the waiting list would either succumb to their disease before receiving a transplant or indeed leave the program to attend heart/lung programs that accessed a larger donor pool. A donor surgical team prepared to travel to other centres to perform the donor extractions would be an essential part of a sustainable program.

I had barely begun to bask in the success the ICU had experienced in dramatically decreasing the wait time from arrival of the donor in Toronto to the OR scheduled time, when Joel was asking me to take on the next step of the donor process. It was past time for us to begin to acquire the donor organs from a distance. This aspect of the program, as everything with Joel, had an urgency about it. Could we start tomorrow? I recognized that my days at the recipient table would end for awhile.

Unfortunately, I took the assignment as a rejection of my contributions to the program and became sullen and withdrawn within the program itself. I would still do the occasional recipient when we were short-handed, but that seemed little compensation. I retreated to the ICU, where I made the decisions and reluctantly began to plan how the donor procedure might come together if undertaken at distant hospitals. I was young and failed to realize that my change in attitude only reflected a lack of a constructive approach to what had been a team effort all along. Instead of recognizing that Joel was giving me operative independence outside the hospital, I internalized the situation in a negative fashion. The realization of the nature of my reaction would not be apparent to me until I returned as head of the program in 1993, and at that time had to undertake the same function of assigning tasks within the surgical side of the program. To Joel's credit, he provided me the appropriate recognition for the achievements we were to make in this area. As time elapsed and the program grew, I came to recognize the importance of a strong and reliable donor acquisition program. You don't always require the front-line attention, but it sure is nice.

Given the urgency exemplified by patients such as Daniel, Joel's request that the distant retrieval program start the next day was understandable. Nonetheless, I had hoped to discuss things with other transplant teams experienced in distant procurement in order to develop an operational plan that would allow us to properly integrate into the process. Before I could bring together the relevant participants, I was informed that there was a lung donor waiting on us in Ottawa. The liver team from London and the kidney team in Ottawa had already indicated their availability. As the new fellows involved in remote "harvesting," we were last-minute add-ons to the entire process, and a time had already been determined for the donor operation to commence. We had yet to work out the logistics of transportation of the surgeons and of preserving and transporting the organ. Yet here was a great opportunity to undertake a distant retrieval fairly close to home. We had a unique opportunity to determine where the glitches might exist within the entire process. As a result, we went unprepared—much as we had done when we first embarked on transplantation. We seemed to have a penchant for doing things on the fly. I could also add that we revelled in it.

Thus it was that I boarded a Lear jet for a trip to Ottawa. It was a jet belonging to a private company. Toronto General had employed such means of transportation in the past for the delivery of patients to our intensive care units from peripheral hospitals and other places quite far afield. Today I don't even recall the name of the recipient that night. I do, however, recall that it was as usual late in the evening.

We arrived at the Ottawa Civic Hospital just before midnight. After examining the patient in the intensive care unit, we proceeded to an old operating theatre. It was very quiet. In fact, I remember that characteristic about almost every operating room I would visit over the next twelve years. They were quiet after hours.

I was sent to Ottawa with a resident assistant and a coordinator by the name of Mel Cohen. Mel was a likable fellow who had been involved in organ donation with the kidney program for several years and now had expanded his role to support the lung program as well. Liver and cardiac transplantation, although well established elsewhere, had not yet been undertaken at TGH. I recall little of the procedure itself. That is probably because my penchant for making notes was attenuated by my sense of relegation to the donor side of the procedure. I do remember fussing over the blood gases and chest x-ray.

Within a year, on subsequent donor forays, the concerns that I expressed with the assessment that night would seem trivial. But this was our first distant retrieval; and thus pragmatic concerns and a tendency towards conservatism on my part were to be expected. Finally I decided that this donor was indeed satisfactory (today we would deem it ideal) and placed a call to Toronto instructing them that they could now anaesthetize the recipient. Considering what still had to be done and our travel time back to Toronto, they should be waiting for me by the time I arrived, thus reducing the ischemic time to a minimum.

As we had not worked out an alternative means of lung preservation, I followed our standard protocols. That involved collapsing the lungs by discontinuing ventilation once the heart had stopped. The chest cavity was then filled with ice-cold saline solution while I waited for the perfusion of stabilizing solutions established by the liver team to be completed. Once they provided an all clear, I removed the heart and the lungs—a much easier technical exercise than the formal separation of the heart from the lungs when both organs are to be utilized in separate recipients. The heart would be removed from its attachments to the lungs once we arrived back in the Toronto General operating room. Having accomplished the removal of the heart and lungs without adverse event, I placed the organs in a sterile plastic bag and handed it all to Mel Cohen. After calling the pilots at the airport to signal our imminent arrival, I went to the change room.

I met Mel at the elevator just outside the operating room suites. He was standing there holding a cardboard box. What struck me as unusual was the fact there was water dripping onto the floor from the seams in the box. To my horror, I realized that the box must contain the lungs and that the ice used to pack them and maintain them at approximately 4 degrees Celsius was rapidly melting.

"Mel," I said, "are the lungs in that thing? It's leaking water all over the place. At this rate, all the ice will be melted before we get to the airport." This was simply not permissible, as once the lungs are allowed to warm, deterioration would occur swiftly.

Mel went on to explain that this was the system they had for shipping the kidneys between hospitals in Toronto. Indeed it was the same box used for the transportation of donor blood, as evidenced by the Red Cross symbols on it. It was actually a standard cardboard box reinforced with Styrofoam™ on the inside for insulation. The latter, however, was not a single piece of moulded Styrofoam but rather consisted of six separate pieces lining each of the sides of the box. The bag containing the lungs was inside and there was ice surrounding the bag. All this was then contained by the Styrofoam liner. The insulating layer of Styrofoam was very thin and the subsequently melting ice was in danger of completely destroying the box.

I had visions of its dissolving in front of us, spilling its rather obvious contents onto the floor to the wonderment of every casual passerby. Visions of the endangered box waiting for the most embarrassing moment to disgorge its contents were paramount. There was the bag of lungs landing with a wet splat on the pavement as we climbed up into the ambulance for the ride to the airport or tumbling down the gangway of the plane onto the tarmac. In each case, of course, I visualized the bag splitting much like the water bombs employed during the heady days of first apartments at University, to be heralded with as much enthusiasm by onlookers as by the unfortunate recipients of our university pranks.

I was convinced that we had to find a solution to this problem before leaving the hospital. We had to ensure that the leakage would stop and that the cold liquid left after the ice melted would at least still be in contact with the lungs rather than dripping incessantly on the floor. Frantic for an answer to our problem, I also recognized that it was now about three a.m., hardly a great time to find assistance in a hospital. A request for a cooler from the nursing staff was likely to receive a less than enthusiastic reception, especially from two unknown characters claiming to be transplant surgeons accompanied by a dripping cardboard box.

At least the operating room nurses would know us, so I ran back and peeked into the operating room. All the nurses were busy assisting both the liver and kidney surgeons in their aspect of the procedure. Before poking my head in the door, I realized that I was now in my street clothes, unsterile, and hence unlikely of a warm reception from those within. Frustrated, I slowly let the operating door slide shut soundlessly and ran back towards their sterile supply area, desperately hoping that something would thrust itself in my path and present itself as the ideal container for our precious cargo. As a surgeon you just come to expect someone to present you with the required equipment. But there was nothing there, either. I walked back through the automatic doors to the elevator. By now there was a sizable puddle around Mel Cohen and the tips of his shoes looked like he had been out in the snow without rubbers. This was becoming too much. We had a plane waiting, not to mention a patient already asleep in another city.

Necessity, they say, is the mother of invention; and necessity guided me back through the doors to the nursing station within the operating room. I knew where the appropriate container had to be—it was always there. And sure enough, it was. Behind the glass partition and under the main operating room desk was the ubiquitous garbage can with an almost empty black garbage bag liner. Worried that someone would appear momentarily and accost me for being in street clothes within the operating room, I moved quickly. Quickly meant dumping the few items in the garbage bag onto the floor. The bag was thus empty save for a small amount of residual coffee spilt from a half-drunk disposable cup. I yelled at Mel to push for the elevator and jumped in with the contraband bag in hand just as the doors were closing.

By the time we arrived at the ground floor, the cardboard box had been unceremoniously stuffed into the bag, one whole sodden side breaking apart in the effort. At the airport we would add a full bag of ice to the garbage bag from the private stores of the pilots to ensure that our temperature was maintained all the way to Toronto General. Relieved, I was asleep before the plane lifted off.

By the time we arrived in Toronto, I was rested and no longer concerned about the preservation of our donor lungs. There was still a considerable amount of ice that could be palpated through the garbage bag. The bag was watertight and too cold to touch for long. We confidently took a police escort to the hospital.

Unfortunately, my embarrassment was not finished for the night. One must appreciate the geography of the second floor at Toronto General. The elevators exit at one end of a large waiting room that serves as the place where the families of patients in the

ICU wait for news of their loved ones. Families of patients undergoing surgery wait elsewhere. However, as the recipient was already in the operating room and as he/she would be going directly to the ICU, the family was indeed waiting there. Unfortunately for me, they were able to recognize me and were perfectly aware of the fact that I had gone off to operate on the donor and that this was to be our first attempt at distant retrieval of the donor lungs. Like many families in the program they were impressed by what they interpreted as very high-tech medicine and surgery. They were about to be disappointed. Unfortunately for me one of them was pacing by the elevator door as it opened and spewed me out accompanied by one bulging and now somewhat moist appearing black garbage bag. I well remember his announcing, "Dr. Todd is here, Dr. Todd is here—they're back!"

There was a rush of dishevelled family members carrying blankets supplied by the nursing staff. Mel and I were surrounded before we could safely get to the corridor doors.

"How did it go? Dr. Cooper told us they were going ahead. Are the lungs good?" or words to that effect were repeated from all of them at once. Then they saw the bag. There were several odd facial expressions shared between them and suddenly there was no one speaking any longer. I actually tried to hide the bag behind my back and stammered out the first phrase that hit me. "Yes, all went very well. The lungs seem fine. Excuse me—I really must get to the OR. We'll be out to talk to you as soon as we are finished." (Of course, I made no notes of that night and my comments may have been somewhat less believable and my exit less dignified.)

I left them speechless and I could hear the faint murmurs of disbelief as I walked away as quickly as I could. In retrospect, I would have been far better off to have coolly responded that all went well and the lungs would be brought to the OR shortly, leaving them to interpret for themselves what odd instruments or equipment would be carried in a standard black garbage bag!

This first expedition into the world of lung retrieval from other centres seemed to set the tenor for the future. In the succeeding years, there would be a number of retrieval adventures. Some were frightening, others outright comical, and of course many became routine. The ones I remember are the two former types. Those are prominent in my mind and will occupy a part of our next chapter.

CHAPTER 8

On the Trail of Donors

Our first foray into distant procurement of donor lungs had proven a success. The lungs brought home in a garbage bag from Ottawa had functioned reasonably well. There had been the usual clinical and radiographic signs of damage from the ischemia (lack of blood supply) itself or possibly from early rejection, but in the end the patient had done well.

However, we still did not understand the root cause of the early lung dysfunction that by this time seemed a routine part of the post-operative course. We had come to accept it as part of the expected phenomena of lung transplantation. We were to learn over the succeeding couple of years that the problem with early malfunction of the donor lungs was in reality a function of our poor efforts at lung preservation. As I have noted elsewhere, it had been our habit from the outset of the program to preserve the lungs simply by collapsing them and immersing them in a cold electrolyte solution. Then after extraction we transported the organs in a bag of cold preservative solution surrounded by copious amounts of ice. At the time, this had appeared to be the most efficient means of achieving the desired result. We knew that the organs needed to be cold to limit their metabolism and hence energy requirements. It seemed that our ability to cool the organ would be enhanced if the lungs were deflated, thus decreasing the surface area. Although not without logic, the procedure flew in the face of every other protocol for ischemic prophylaxis developed by transplant teams for liver, heart, and kidney.

In each of these latter instances, it was common practice to insert catheters into the artery supplying the organ prior to the arrest of the circulation. Then as the blood pressure began to fall dramatically from the interventions of the surgeons, the infusion of a cold preservative solution directly into the organs' blood vessels would be commenced. This would take some ten to twenty minutes until the prescribed volume had been attained.

In the mid-1980s we were the only ones performing lung transplants and thus had come to assume that the impaired early function of the transplanted lung was a constant; something predictable and to be expected.

Thus, in 1986, it was commonplace for our recipients to spend several days to a few weeks in the intensive care unit and to require mechanical ventilation for at least five to seven days while the new lung recovered from the insult. We presumed that this would be the norm, as there was no other program for comparison. We wrongly assumed that this was standard fare and that there was little we could do about the situation. We were as blind to the problem with donors as our predecessors had been with the recipient operation and the post-operative management. All our early efforts had been expended on the care of the recipient. True, we had defined the criteria for donor selection that in our minds seemed appropriate. However, our concern and thought about the donor stopped there.

We cannot even take credit for initiating the evolution in the methods for donor lung preservation. In reality it was through the advice of the cardiac and liver surgeons that we modified our extraction techniques to employ a perfusion system. As I have noted, such was the mainstay of their preservation technique.

We had already discovered that the distant extractions frequently involved multiple teams from all over North America. At each of these it was abundantly clear that we alone did not employ perfusion systems. Moreover, we found ourselves waiting to commence the actual extraction process following the initial dissection due to the fact that their preservatives were flowing. Clearly, our adoption of a similar technique would not delay the procedure at all, and our colleagues suggested this might actually improve early lung performance. Indeed it did.

This was to dramatically alter the immediate post-operative lung function. Within a short time following the initiation of donor lung perfusion prior to extraction, we recorded a significant decrease in the number of days of required ventilatory support. By 1990 it would become commonplace for our patients to be weaned from the ventilator within hours of their surgery and to spend no longer than two to three days in the intensive care unit. This was a far cry from our early experience wherein the patients had been in the intensive care unit for weeks at a time and had frequently returned for further ventilator assistance. Brief stays in the intensive care unit were not routine, of course. There remained those patients who, despite all our efforts to reduce ischemic times and provide for maximum protection with the infusion of various preservative solutions, still experienced signs of significant lung damage that precluded an early wean from the ventilator.

There was one other hurdle to overcome. It was considered impossible to provide both a heart and a lung from the same donor, simply because both surgical teams wanted some of the same tissue. The arteries and veins between the heart and lungs are short. Both teams required sufficient length to adequately and safely perform their subsequent implantations. The perceived inability to utilize the same donor greatly impeded our access to lungs. There were always cardiac recipients desperately in need of a heart, with only days or weeks to live if our lung recipient took the donor. We therefore had to come up with a way to provide a heart and lung from the same donor. Thus we invited cardiac surgeons from Ottawa and London, the two cardiac transplant sites in Ontario, to attend our autopsy suite where we proposed to demonstrate the technique we had worked out to accomplish this objective. Although skeptical that such a procedure could provide them with satisfaction, cardiac surgeons from the two Ontario programs were willing to attend. As they were our major competitors for the donor, this was the place to start.

At our meeting in the autopsy suite of Toronto General Hospital, we pointed out how a single donor could provide organs for two or three recipients—one heart and two lungs. The lungs could be utilized for a single recipient for a double lung transplant or alternatively could be placed as single transplants in two separate patients. Thus from one donor there was the opportunity to provide a transplanted organ for three waiting patients. Initiating this as an action plan would, however, depend on our ability that day to convince our out-of-town colleagues that such was feasible. Their immediate response to the suggestion was predictable and swift: "It can't be done."

This we were anticipating. Over the phone or in a conference room, further discussion would have been impossible. But here in the autopsy suite there was nothing to lose. The technical curiosity of each surgeon was piqued. Whether they just wanted to see us fail miserably—hence putting the issue to rest—or whether they were intrigued by the description of what we wished to show them was of no concern to us at the time. What we wanted was their undivided and hopefully unbiased attention. One of the surgeons stated that he would leave early for home, but the other was reasonable and sufficiently curious to encourage him to stay. As I said to them: "You've come all this way—why don't you let us show you what we suggest?"

Naturally, Joel Cooper and I had worked out the actual surgical technique during a previous session. Thus there was little surprise when they acknowledged that it could certainly be achieved in the autopsy suite. Although recognizing feasibility in the autopsy dissection, they emphasized that performing it on a beating heart would present different challenges. Any further reservation, however, was removed by our suggestion that we try this together when the next appropriate donor presented him/herself; and if successful, develop a collaborative paper on the technique for publication.

The offer of a collaborative publication that would enhance everyone's curriculum vitae provided the final persuasion if indeed anything further was required. With their agreement to proceed with separate lung and heart donation from the same donor, the way was cleared for our access to the entire Canadian donor pool. However, we would never be capable of acquiring the same numbers as the liver and cardiac programs. The simple truth was that lungs deteriorate quickly once brain death has occurred. We would learn that at the best of times we might anticipate accepting only twenty percent of the donors offered to our program.

On the other hand, the total number of available donors in the province was soon to increase. This was largely due to the development of a centralized agency for the identification and distribution of donor organs. The effort of individual hospitals was to be replaced by an agency called MORE—an acronym for Multiple Organ Retrieval and Exchange. Prior to the birth of MORE, the only hospitals with an internal organization geared to identify organ donors and secure consent were those actively involved in transplantation. MORE would expand this responsibility throughout the province of Ontario and provide a template for the other provinces.

It wasn't long before there was a national system of interactive agencies. By the late nineteen eighties, Canada possessed the ability to place a donor in Vancouver to the most seriously ill patient on the other side of the country. This was accomplished through the co-operation of the transplant surgeons across the country. They agreed upon priority definitions that provided guidance to the provincial agencies so that everyone was aware of the list of potential recipients for each organ system. In addition, all possessed a clear understanding of the rank order of priority for each patient. In essence there developed a co-operative program of data sharing that ensured as best as possible that no organs were lost due to inefficiencies or a lack of knowledge. Each province retained its own right of first refusal for even a lower priority patient, but once it was determined that a particular province could not utilize the organ in question, the national matching system would be activated. In addition, an extremely urgent requirement could now be advertised nationally and thus could override the particular province's own priorities.

The obsession to attempt to place every single donor organ was nurtured by the constant reminder that some of our potential recipients would succumb to their disease without ever having had the opportunity of a transplant. This one fact frequently could create a moral dilemma for the transplant surgeon, and such became a frequent occurrence in Toronto as the program expanded and the physician resource base dwindled.

In that regard, it is important to remember that donors appear with no predictability. In the lung program, several weeks could pass without a single donor. There might be several calls that managed to extract you from your bed, but these did not always translate into a transplant. This might be followed by a rapid succession of usable donors over a short time period. I recall performing three or four transplants in a single week— sometimes two in twenty-four hours or three in seventy-two hours. That may not seem to be onerous, but remember that the transplants constituted additional activity to an already full surgical practice. They also had the predilection to occur at night. Thus one would finish the normal day of ten to twelve hours only to engage in several calls from the MORE coordinator while one determined if the donor was suitable. This would be followed by the procedure itself, which for the donor team could take from four to ten hours, depending on how far one had to travel.

Once MORE became involved, it became more difficult in the middle of night to refuse the offered donor because of fatigue or the concern to preserve your operative list for the next day. I recall many nights conversing with the MORE coordinator, wishing that there would be some specific problem with this donor that would provide the legitimate excuse to permit me to decline the offer and go back to sleep. A surgical ego would never accommodate the admission that perhaps your surgical judgment and operative skills might be impaired by the lack of sleep. Pride was better served by an apparent problem with the donor. These were times when fatigue was deep.

A further moral dilemma was created by the fact that a transplant frequently resulted in the cancellation of a previously booked surgery. The surgical list for us usually consisted of patients with cancer of the intra-thoracic organs. As the waiting lists for such patients grew long in the 1990s, the decisions became increasingly painful. The transplant might proceed, but your patient with lung cancer who has waited eight weeks for his/her surgery was to be cancelled. More than once I can remember the incredulous voice of the coordinator: "You're turning down this donor? But it's perfect for Mary X!"

There were times after hanging up the phone that the voice of guilt in your mind was simply too strident to permit sleep to return. Then you'd call back and hope that no one else had claimed the lung. If you weren't about to be able to regain some rest then you might as well be in the operating room. Making choices between patients is never pleasant.

Once MORE became a reality, the assessment of donors and the matching with the most critical recipients became an external function. The algorithms at least permitted the coordinators to exclude some donors without contacting us. Prior to that, however, the number of spurious calls received was even more significant. Nonetheless, within the pulmonary transplant program we could anticipate four or five calls for every donor lung that we eventually retrieved. The impact of these calls was notable, as the process of donor acquisition is protracted and extends far beyond the operative procedure and the travel time required. There are a number of assessments that must be made to ensure that the potential donor is appropriate in general terms, and then a whole series of specific tests for each organ system to ensure that it is functional and is compatible with a specific recipient.

The coordinator arranges for the performance of several blood tests and radiological examinations designed to determine suitability. In particular, AIDS and hepatitis blood tests are performed to ensure that disease is not transmitted. Unfortunately, the HIV (AIDS) test could sometimes take twenty-four hours and the transplants usually will have taken place by the time the test is finalized.

During my years at Toronto General I recall but one case where the donor tested positive for AIDS. Clearly if there is a clinical suspicion that the donor is at high risk for the disease, the procedure would be placed on hold until the test results are known. I have certainly insisted on that several times. However, in many cases it becomes a matter of either rejecting the donor or performing the procedure without the test result, as the donor and/or one or more organ systems will deteriorate quickly after brain death is declared. With the full knowledge that the intended recipient(s) may never get a second chance at a donor, these decisions were not made lightly.

I would be contacted when a coordinator determined that a patient on my waiting list was appropriate for a given donor. Because the Toronto lung program was the busiest in the country even after the other centres became active, we would often be offered donor lungs from afar irrespective of the priority rating. It was not unusual for there to be several patients on our list with the same blood type and priority. It would be my job at that point to determine which one would receive the lungs. Sometimes this was not an easy decision. Once I had made that decision, the coordinator would inform me of the chest x-ray findings and the donor's arterial blood gases (the content of oxygen and carbon dioxide in the blood stream).

We had determined in the early eighties what would be our lower limit of acceptable oxygenation in the donor. Such should reflect the functionality of the lung to be transplanted. As time passed and our experience grew, we began gradually to consider acceptance of lower limits. Our lower limit initially was 300 millimetres of mercury (I believe it is the same today). However, what do you do if the value is 295 mm? Well, if you haven't seen a donor for awhile and the intended recipient is critical, you say yes and trust that the previously determined limits are as arbitrary as you know them to be. Then once you have decided that the difference of 5 mm of mercury had no dire consequences, you're primed to consider the donor with a value of 290 when the circumstances again present a recipient who may never be provided with another opportunity.

Thus it is a bit of a balancing act. In practice, if the value was below 300 I would request therapeutic interventions to improve things with a repeat of the test in another hour or two. If the value was well over 300 and everything else seemed fine I would still ask for the test to be repeated at intervals. We were all very much aware of the fact that the extent of oxygenation could change dramatically and rapidly once brain death ensued. Thus it was imperative to be certain that oxygenation was maintained while we waited for the arrangements to be completed. I have seen values of 450 fall precipitously to less than 100 in a matter of an hour or less. Thus the stage is set for numerous calls before we finally arrive at the airport. Adding to the complexity is the fact that the other transplant programs may be agitating to complete the process and proceed as quickly as possible. Certainly I have found myself on that side of the fence on several occasions and needed to remind myself of the concerns that I might have if placed in the same situation. In the end, however, each program recognizes its responsibilities to patients within its own program.

The passage of time brings with it physiological alterations in the donor. Indeed, following brain death, cardiac and pulmonary dysfunction are common, usually resulting in the onset of cardiac standstill within forty-eight to seventy-two hours. The abnormal physiology is not entirely understood, and there remain some aspects of this dysfunction that are obscure. For example, even in a young brain-dead victim, cardiac failure can occur without any demonstrable physical lesion seen in the heart at autopsy. As a result, cardiac function is assessed carefully before donation and there are occasions when the lungs can be utilized but the heart cannot, due to impaired contractile function.

As a consequence of these numerous alterations in heart and lung function, the first phone call from the coordinator is followed by many more over the next several hours. There are calls concerning the response to therapy in an effort to correct the oxygen levels, calls to inform us that one of the transplant teams is delayed, calls to tell us that blood pressure is now unstable and do we have suggestions for the donor hospital physicians, calls to tell us that our operating rooms are full of emergencies and could we please delay for a few more hours. The calls seem endless and as they almost always occur late at night, provide a constant interruption of any attempt to gain some rest.

I've talked about the problem of sleep deprivation before and would not want the reader to assume that this is another physician placing his own comforts ahead of the patient's requirements. Our rest is crucial, as shortly we will be expected to perform at our peak for several hours, after we have already participated in a full surgical day. Since so often the initial call came after we had retired to bed for the night, I was in the habit of taking the first call in the family room. Then I would lie down on the couch with a portable phone beside me to attend to the myriad other calls until it was time to leave for the airport. At least that way I could pick up the phone on the first ring and the subsequent conversation was not disruptive to the entire household. Otherwise, to protect their own sleep, my family may have ensured that the locks on the doors were changed before I returned!

Sleep always returned quickly after a call but was rarely satisfying. The mind remains active anticipating the next call or the ring of the alarm. As I was usually in the downstairs of the house, I would often ask the coordinator to play the role of the alarm and call me in sufficient time to enable me to drive to the airport. So many times with marginal donors, I would field seven or eight calls throughout the night only to have determined that the donor was not suitable. But the job didn't end there. The operating room, ICU, and other surgeons all had to be notified as well. By the time we would be finished for the night another three or four calls would be necessary. I could only hope that there was sufficient time for a little sleep before the day would start again in earnest.

There were several times that the donor would prove problematic and all arrangements were cancelled. Unfortunately, I might not return to the comfort of a real bed and its attendant alarm clock, preferring the immediacy of the couch. I would then be awakened in the morning by my wife with the realization that the day was not only going to be tiring but tardy as well.

Between calls, the coordinator arranged the flights or at times a limousine or ambulance if the donor hospital was nearby. The hospital had access to private company jets that could be responsive to our arbitrary departure times. It is hard to find a commercial flight leaving at 0200 hours for Sudbury or Ottawa. The aircrew was accustomed to providing service for businessmen and thus we at least could be certain of having some sort of food and beverage on board. If we couldn't sleep, at least we could eat.

Unfortunately, not all aircraft were of this calibre. There were several flights in unheated, turboprop aircraft that seemed to bob and weave and generally lurch about in a discordant fashion. For the nervous flyer, this led to the inescapable conclusion that the surgeon was about to become the next donor. In fact, at one point in order to cut costs, these less-spectacular aircraft that were apparently at the disposal of the provincial government became routine for the shorter flights. The noise level and uneven ride was so disruptive at a time when one was attempting to find a place of calm before the real action began, a formal objection was made that resulted in a return to the non-governmental aircraft. In fact it took the refusal of one of the transplant surgeons to board the plane that resulted in a reversal of this economization.

At our destination, we would usually be met by an ambulance or police vehicle to facilitate transportation to the appropriate hospital. The same would be true upon our return to Toronto. At the Toronto end, the mode of transportation was in the beginning exclusively police escort. This appeared to be an activity they greatly enjoyed and I can only speak in complimentary terms of their co-operation and goodwill. Indeed, these encounters found me expressing new respect for the Toronto Police. Those fellows really know how to drive. It was apparent that they greatly relished the opportunity to demonstrate their skill behind the wheel.

As I have noted elsewhere, the early days of lung transplantation found us deeply concerned with the length of ischemic time. We had communicated to the police the necessity for rapid transit from Pearson International Airport to the hospital. We sincerely believed that a reduction in transportation time of several minutes would be beneficial. Logic, however, would dictate that a decrease in travel time from the airport of ten minutes would hardly be important. Yet it took some time for the obvious to become a practical reality. In part I am convinced that was because we truly enjoyed the excitement of the police cars dashing through traffic with sirens wailing and lights flashing.

To be sure, we were impatient as well, and anything that would provide a quick fix to Toronto traffic was indeed welcome. In time the police chase cars would be replaced with ambulance transport. At least we would still have the option of sirens and lights to ensure ready access through congested motorways should we arrive during the rush-hour peaks. But for some time, the police were our partners in flight. I simply revelled in their skill and greatly enjoyed hurtling down the road at 160 km/hr against oncoming traffic, dodging the approaching cars. It was especially exhilarating to watch the horrified faces of the drivers and passengers in the oncoming vehicles. I always had the front passenger's seat, since it became clear early on that my partners in the donor retrieval process did not share my perceptions of what constituted fun in a car. This seemed abundantly fair, as I was definitely not enamoured of plane rides, so the others deserved a period of discomfort in compensation.

After stowing the cooler containing the lung and our bags of equipment in the trunk of the car, I would slip into the front passenger's seat by default, as no one else wished to sit there. The police driver would always turn to me with a hopeful grin on his face and ask:

"Are we in a hurry, Doc?"

"Of course!" I would reply.

"Bells and whistles, then?" would be the retort.

"Bells and whistles it is!" I would say. The conversation was always the same. It was accompanied by a collective groan from my colleagues in the back seat. On every occasion, the officer would provide the kind of magnificent smile that one sees when newly made fathers first observe their offspring or the family greets the long-absent loved one at the airport. It was a grin that was truly infectious, full of mirth and anticipation. It expressed delight and at the same time beamed a challenge across the space between us that seemed to say—"Are you ready for this?" The smile would be accompanied by a practised removal of his hat onto the seat between us. They consistently did that. I'm not sure how the removal of their hat facilitated their anticipated wild driving but it was constant and a sure sign of a fast-paced approach to our transport. So common was this that I remember an occasion when I had verified the bells and whistles approach to our ride out of earshot from my colleagues. As they entered the rear seat, one of them noted that the officer had his hat off and exclaimed: "Oh, oh—it's one of those!"

Toronto's main throughways can become gridlocked with only minor increases in volume or trivial accidents, since the baseline volume of traffic dictates that the roads rapidly approach the marginal limits of functionality. Hence there were many wild rides. I recall riding at speeds in excess of 160 kph on the shoulder of highway ramps, charging headlong into the approaching traffic, and weaving back and forth in multi-laned roadways from outside to inside with abandon.

On one occasion, there were two cars waiting for us, as we had visitors from other programs along on an educational exercise. We clearly required additional space, and as usual the police were accommodating. It was early in the morning in Toronto and the highways were solid. I was in the second car, desperately wishing I were watching the action in the lead vehicle. As we sped along the Gardiner Expressway in the passing lane, the cars occupying that lane responded to the sirens and lights by entering the adjacent right lane. Some responded quickly, while others were somnolent and had slow reaction times. Thus the police drivers had to be especially alert and moderate their speed so that they didn't play bumper cars with the slow responders—a manoeuvre that I think would have pleased them greatly had it been within the bounds of their permitted acts.

At the Kingsway intersection, I saw the car in front of our lead vehicle pull over as anticipated. Both the lead police vehicle and the one I occupied surged ahead. However, the civilian driver failed to note that there were *two* police vehicles and made a hasty effort to regain his position in the left lane. Meanwhile, our driver had commenced his rather rapid acceleration to the point where indeed we seemed about to go up and over this unfortunate fellow who now occupied the space in front of us. Undaunted, the officer did not brake the car but in one fluid movement restarted the sirens and squeezed to the right into an impossibly small space just vacated a moment ago by the somnolent fellow who was the subject of his frustration. He followed this by a sideways slide back into the left lane that would have done the movie industry proud. I was amazed and this time wondered about the advisability of our haste. My friends were not pleased. The officer had a grin that portrayed nothing short of sheer joy. He didn't even comment. I did, however, interject with an appropriate compliment; afterwards assuring my colleagues that it was not intended to provide encouragement.

I recall the last time we utilized the police as an escort to the hospital in Toronto. We had flown to Ottawa to obtain the lungs from an unfortunate victim of a cerebral vascular hemorrhage. The intended recipient was a teenager. This young man had been on the program for some time, as his blood group was not common. The latter circumstance precluded his allocation of the majority of donors. This was a young person who had rapidly endeared himself to the members of the program, both medical personnel and patients alike. Not only was Jason a handsome and pleasant young man, but he was at all times much like Cameron, whose story was depicted in Chapter 3.

Never demanding, continually positive, he was a well-thought-of individual. Like Cameron, he appeared mature beyond his years and, despite the terminal nature of his illness, accepted his fate and the perilous path that was required to secure his future. As time passed without the appearance of a donor of the same blood type who approximated his size, he became a regular subject of discussion within the team. Once again, we considered utilizing a less than ideal donor in order to provide him with an opportunity to survive. The donor in Ottawa that afternoon, however, appeared ideal, and we were all excited and positive that at last we would be able to assist this young man. For once this was to be an afternoon excursion with a real chance that the entire procedure might be completed by midnight.

We flew to Ottawa in one of the leased private company jets, and I remember commenting as we boarded in Toronto that this plane was extremely well appointed, with plush leather seats that were wider than usual, fancy pot lights in the ceiling, and considerable more room than the standard Lear Jet. The pilot, with whom I had flown before, informed me that this was an entirely different plane. Today the name of the jet has vanished in the depths of my memory banks but suffice it to say it was very nice. As you will see, it was extremely well outfitted.

Feeling properly pampered, our buoyant spirits were rudely dampened upon arrival at the Civic hospital. This was the same hospital that had been the site of our first attempt at distant retrieval. I recalled for my resident who had accompanied me, the incident with the garbage bag, never realizing that I was again about to embarrass myself. Upon our arrival, we were informed that the oxygenation of the donor had been falling steadily since our departure from Toronto. The donor was now in the operating room and the liver team from Montreal had already commenced the procedure. Once we entered the room and were scrubbed and gowned, they graciously stepped back from the table to permit us to examine the lungs. I did note, however, that the surgeon in charge of the liver team seemed somewhat irritated at being displaced, even if this was an expected part of the operation.

The anaesthetist had already informed me that the oxygen level had fallen to 280 mm Hg (recall that our lowest acceptable value was 300). However, I had determined that I would be willing to accept a lower oxygen level, given the difficulty in obtaining a donor for this young man. If the lungs appeared normal, then we would take the chance for him. After opening the breast bone, I accessed both sides of the chest cavity and the lungs eagerly herniated forth into the operative field. They were over-expanded and looked very normal. My resident commented that they looked pink and perfect. However, what is seen initially through the incision in the sternum is the anterior or front portion of the lungs, largely composed of the upper or superior lobes. One has to actually manually deliver the dependent or lower lobes forward into the operative field. To our great disappointment, these were abnormal on both sides. They both were discoloured and poorly inflated, causing us to wonder about early infection. Even with pressure exerted by the anaesthetist, they would not properly expand again, suggesting that they were stiff and non-compliant.

Despite their appearance, I remained committed to securing these lungs. I scrubbed out and went to the nurses' station to discuss things with the rest of the team in Toronto in an attempt to share the responsibility for what I was about to propose. The Montreal surgeon was less than pleased that I was delaying his operation and grunted at me to be quick about it. Given the circumstances, the recipient team in Toronto immediately agreed that this course of action was best.

I returned to the room determined that we would make this work. I stuck my head into the room to announce that we would proceed and to let them all know that I was about to re-scrub. Given the impatience of the liver team, I was moving to the scrub sink before finishing my sentence. Thus I only vaguely heard them call my name as the door swung closed. However this was to be followed quickly by a nurse who informed me that my resident wanted further discussion before I scrubbed.

Indeed he did, and rightly so. Oxygenation had deteriorated further. The last test sent by the anaesthetist revealed an oxygen level of only 210 mm Hg. Dismayed by the absolute value, I was also distressed by the rapidity of its decline. Past experience had taught me that such was always associated with severely damaged lungs. The only other possibility was an unrecognized obstruction to airflow in the trachea or bronchi. Since we had come this far, it seemed reasonable to make sure, and I requested a bronchoscope to examine the airways. As I waited for the bronchoscope to arrive, the anaesthetist decided to send another test just in case the last one had been erroneous. The result returned just as I verified that the airways were patent and normal. It was now 170mm. Hg. The other teams by this time were more than anxious to get under way and complete their extractions before oxygenation deteriorated to the point where blood pressure itself would become problematic.

"Are you going ahead or not?" the liver surgeon from Montreal asked with obvious irritation in his voice.

I thought for a minute of Jason and of Cameron who had died several years before. I desperately wanted to return to Toronto with good news for the former, having never been able to deliver such for the latter.

"No," I said. "Get on with what you have to do. Sorry to take so long. Our recipient is an AB blood type."

I didn't have to say anything more. The others immediately recognized why we were distressed and understood the motivation behind our attempt to push the envelope. The Montreal surgeon looked over the top of his mask with much softer eyes and as if to remedy his previous remarks said:

"OK. I understand, no problem. Good luck and fly home safely."

On the trip back to the airport, my resident and I managed to work ourselves into a state of decided unhappiness at the misfortune that had occurred. Recognizing that this may well have been the last chance that this young man would have to acquire new lungs, neither of us was anxious to return home and break the news to him. As I recall, the entire issue was aggravated by the fact that it had been a week of disastrous complications on the Thoracic Service. This latest tragedy served to remind us of our unproductive week and of our own ineptitude as surgical saviours. By the time we reached the Ottawa private aerodrome, our mood was unpleasant.

The pilots were incredulous at our early arrival and somewhat disappointed as they had already settled in to watch a movie in the lounge reserved for VIP passengers. One look at our faces was sufficient to tell them that the news was not the best; and if that failed to convince them, our less than friendly responses quickly quashed the usual casual banter that we commonly enjoyed with them on such occasions. We had flown with these fellows before. They understood the process that was involved and appreciated the fact that we were dealing with real people and not hypothetical realities. We enjoyed an excellent rapport. Thus they commiserated with our distress.

My resident roughly tossed the equipment bags into the back of the aircraft. The MORE coordinator literally threw the empty cooler onto the plane. Normally it was quite heavy due to the quantity of ice packed around the organs that were to return to Toronto. I believe that there were some rather expressive adjectives applied to it as it tumbled back down the retractable steps onto the tarmac. Indeed, I recall that adjectives of the four-letter variety were readily and frequently applied to all subjects of our conversation. It was a colourful boarding, and the agitation of the conversation did not improve during takeoff.

As we gained altitude, the co-pilot looked back over his shoulder out of the cockpit and announced that he had just the right answer to our woes. As we had observed already, this was a finely appointed aircraft. Indeed, it was so well stocked that there was a hidden bar at the rear. At his invitation, I explored the richness of its interior to find some really quite nice single malt scotch whisky. Given our mood, this did seem to be the appropriate medication and we managed to treat ourselves to its bounty. In fact, it was such a wonderful idea that we concluded a second round would be an essential part of the remedy. Not being our own scotch, little heed was paid to the quantities dispensed and we were relishing our third when we touched down in Toronto. As we approached the hangar, I noted that there was a police car apparently awaiting our arrival. Turning to the MORE coordinator I asked, "Did you forget to cancel the cop car?"

The look on his face verified what was already obvious. I immediately began to compose my apology and wondered what this might do to the relationship we enjoyed with these fast-driving constables. It then occurred to me that without them we did not have the means to return to the hospital where our cars were parked. Even if a car were available, none of us was at this point in any shape to drive. The answer to our dilemma thus became rather obvious, aided no doubt by the fantastic libations provided by our friends the pilots. They were the only ones who knew that the cooler was empty.

Coming off the airplane, my resident and I "struggled" with the apparently very heavy cooler. We shrugged off the cop's offer of assistance and just asked him to open his trunk. With a great effort we managed to hoist it up and gingerly lay it on the floor of the trunk.

"Good trip?" the officer asked.

"Yup—no problems," I replied. "Hope you haven't been waiting long. I guess you know we're going to Toronto General?"

"Yeah, that's what dispatch said," he answered as he slipped into the driver's seat.

I took my usual place in the front beside the officer. I could sense the tension from my compatriots in the rear when he turned to me and asked;

"Do you want the usual—bells and whistles?"

Again it was no doubt that wonderful scotch that emboldened me to reply, "Yeah, for sure—bells and whistles!" Or perhaps it was just the desire to get the trip over with quickly.

Off came the hat and we were away, successful in our deceit. We bade him farewell at the emergency entrance and continued our charade of struggling with the cooler until he drove away. He gave us a great ride that day. Unless he reads this some day, he will never know that the cooler was empty and he managed to provide police escort to three young men who were half tanked. That was our last trip with the police. Sober minds in the new day determined that we were becoming somewhat cavalier in our approach to the element of time. In the future, we would have occasional rides in the back of an ambulance, but in the end, as time became less of a factor, even that was replaced by our own MORE van. The rides became distinctly more tame.

Jason would wait another while before a donor was available. As happens with recipients who have waited too long and have little time left, a compromised donor was accepted. We could not let this one pass. It was indeed compromised and Jason died of respiratory failure in the early post-operative period. We had seen it coming months before on the way home from Ottawa.

Prior to 1987, we had performed only single lung transplants. There remained a number of clinical conditions for which such an operation was inappropriate. Cystic fibrosis and other varieties of chronic pulmonary infections posed theoretical problems to such an operation. The single lung transplant would of course leave an infected native lung on the other side. The remaining native lung would be a constant source of infection for the patient. Magnified by the requirement of post-operative immunosuppression, such episodes of infection would almost certainly prove life threatening. A successful transplant in such a patient must therefore entail either the removal of the other lung and/or its replacement.

As the disease is congenital, patients with cystic fibrosis are young. The condition is not uncommon, and prior to the emergence of more powerful antibiotics, it often resulted in the demise of patients as young as teenagers. Although in the 1990s some patients with the disease survived well into their fourth decade, it remained universally fatal at some point, as the majority of cystic patients develop respiratory failure by age thirty. As well, there remained a large number with significant respiratory impairment before the age of twenty.

There was thus a clear need to provide some form of lung replacement, and this prospect led the team to consider how we might accomplish a double lung transplant. Until this time, such patients were managed with a heart/lung transplant. Not only did this prevent the utilization of the heart in another separate potential recipient, it also provided a donor heart to a patient who simply did not require one. The patient's heart was perfectly normal, and usually of better quality than the one transplanted. The donor heart would be more appropriately placed in yet another recipient dying of isolated cardiac disease.

As a result, Alec Patterson had been experimenting in Joel's laboratory with a variety of techniques for performing a double lung transplant. Today such an operation is routine and the techniques employed vastly different from that engineered by Alec and his research fellows in the mid-1980s in animal models. When they were ready to share the technique with us, the single lung program was an established success and we were all eager for the next challenge. Although our first surgical technique was awkward, it did work, and by 1986 we were ready to undertake the procedure in something other than laboratory animals.

The subject was Ann Harrison. She had a form of lung disease similar to emphysema but with an infectious component. Like all our other patients, she was entering the terminal stages of her disease. She reminded me greatly of Tom Hall. She was focused and expressed the same confidence that Tom had exhibited three years previously. She was emotionally and physiologically an ideal candidate.

I would perform the donor extraction. We had determined in advance that we would wait for a circumstance when the heart would not be allocated. In that case we could afford to take our time with the extraction. Should we encounter technical errors and difficulties in the separation of heart and lungs according to the laboratory protocol, no harm would be done to a potential cardiac recipient. This seemed wise. I was about to find out just how wise that decision really was.

The donor was eventually found at the Kingston General Hospital. It was a fall evening with heavy rain and strong winds. I had originally been told that we would travel by a fixed-wing turbo-prop airplane and was delighted upon arrival at Pearson airport to discover that a Lear Jet was waiting. My initial enthusiasm was somewhat dampened when the pilot commented that jets did not normally land at Kingston, as the runway was a little too short; and in fact he was rather looking forward to the trip since he had never flown a jet into Kingston. The grin on his face reminded me of our friends in the Provincial Police happily placing their hats on the seat beside them. Such did nothing to quell the steadily increasing anxiety that now firmly had me in its grip.

It was a bumpy but fortunately short flight to Kingston, highlighted literally by bolts of lightening that would abruptly illuminate the interior of the plane. I was already anticipating a quick end to the ordeal when the pilot commenced his descent. Descent does not adequately describe the approach. Abrupt fall from the sky is better. The latter was culminated by several sudden down and up drafts accompanied by a pronounced waggle of the wings. The "Whoa, baby!" from the co-pilot was an encouraging extra touch.

We hit the tarmac with something akin to a thud and then managed to make like a car skidding in the snow as the pilot hit the brakes with a force that flung us against the restraints of the seat belt. I was by now beginning to more adequately understand my colleagues' aversion to the police car rides and was convinced that the pilot was one in disguise. My impressions were confirmed when, on successfully coming to a stop, he yelled back to us

"Wow! Wasn't that great!" I wondered if I could operate with any skill whatsoever with the return trip on my mind.

By the time we reached the hospital, the patient was in the operating room and the abdomen had already been opened by the liver surgeons from Montreal. I was introduced to the nursing and anaesthesia staff in the room and to an extremely keen and interested medical student from Queen's. Queen's University was my alma mater. As other Canadian university graduates will testify, Queen's graduates are insufferable when exposed to their own kind or asked to comment on the quality of their educational experience. We all know it is simply second to none and are anxious to ensure that all others are made painfully aware of this fact. Thus, I was eager to provide this young fellow with an experience to remember and encouraged him to stand as close as he could on a stool to adequately observe the procedure. By the time I arrived at the operating room table scrubbed and gowned, I ensured that he had received full details of the history of transplantation as well as the entire outline of the procedure he was about to witness. Thanks to the Lear Jet pilot my nervous energy was high.

After splitting the sternum, I proceeded to open both pleural spaces (the cavity in the chest containing the lungs), starting with the right side. The right lung looked superb, and, as oxygenation was excellent, I mused that this was all coming together rather nicely. However, the left pleural space was difficult to find. There just did not seem to be a free space between the inside of the chest cavity and the lung. Remember that the lungs reside inside the rigid box of the rib cage. There are normally no attachments between the lungs and the inside of the ribs. It is literally a cavity. Yet in this case there appeared to be dense adhesions between the lung and the inner surface of the cavity. There was no free space.

The donor was nineteen years old. It seemed very unlikely that at that tender age he would have had a disease process that would have resulted in such extensive adhesions between the lung and the chest wall. If indeed the adhesions occupied the entire space, the extraction of the lung would become not only tedious but would carry with it a significant risk of damaging the lung on that side. As my frustration and alarm heightened, I expressed my utter surprise that such a problem would be present in one so young.

"I just don't understand it," I said to my resident on the other side of the table. He must have had tuberculosis or a severe pneumonia as a child, I thought. "Let me see that x-ray again."

The chest x-ray was indeed perfectly clear. There was nothing to suggest a problem with the left lung. As I was again bemoaning the situation I heard the voice of the medical student behind me timidly asking, "Is it possibly related to the operation he had on his left lung?"

"He had a *what*?" I said as I turned my entire frustration onto the coordinator. "You never told me that this guy had had surgery!"

The MORE coordinator is the one with all the information. They process it all and pass the relevant features on to each transplant surgeon. My question was delivered in a brusque and unkind manner, since we all were aware that previous chest surgery in the donor precluded the use of the lungs.

"Tom," he anxiously replied, "no one told me about this—I swear."

Turning from the table to the student, I said as calmly as I could (it probably wasn't all that calm): "So . . . what surgery did this guy have and when?'

"Well, I admitted him to the ICU, and the family said that he had had a tumour removed from his left chest when he was just twelve years old," he replied.

Now my anxiety reached a new level. A previous operation was a relatively strong contraindication to the donor because of the concerns with adhesions. A *tumour*, however, took the problem to an entirely different level. If the tumour had been malignant, then an absolute contraindication existed. One simply would not take the chance of transplanting tumour cells into a recipient who was about to be immuno-suppressed. I quickly tore off my gloves and ran out into the corridor heading for the main OR desk so that I could call Toronto and hopefully stop the recipient operation. I had already indicated that a preliminary check of the donor was positive. I hoped that Joel would not have started the procedure in Toronto without hearing my final confirmation on directly inspecting the lungs. Nonetheless we did not have a specific "failsafe" mechanism for such an eventuality. It was possible that he might have proceeded with the anaesthetic but surely they had not started the actual recipient operation.

"Dr. Cooper can't come to the phone, Dr Todd." The nurse at the TGH operating room desk answered to my request.

"Well, put me through to the room, then," I replied.

"But Dr. Todd, he's started the case. He's scrubbed," she said.

I presumed she meant that the anaesthesia had started and he was standing by. However, the nurse in the room immediately informed me that he could not come to the phone because he was indeed scrubbed and had commenced his incision. There was little more to say. We were now committed. Joel did speak with me aided by the nurse holding the phone to his ear. But there was nothing that could change the course of our activities at this point. I had to go back and do what I could to extract the left lung without too much damage. More important, we had to hope that the tumour had been benign.

People and the systems they create are fallible. This would not be the last time that an error in communication would bring with it the potential for an adverse outcome. As I write this, I am aware of the recent unfortunate incident at a southern university in the United States. Within their thoracic transplant program, a young woman received a heart/lung transplant from a patient of dissimilar blood type. The ensuing complications resulted in significant brain damage. She was declared brain dead and removed from life support systems.

The press speculated on the source of such an error in communication, and all the details will likely remain unavailable.

Although one may never fully understand how such a mistake occurred, I can think of several scenarios that might have led to this unfortunate circumstance. As we have noted, transplantation is an exhausting area of surgical expertise and there are few such individuals in any institution. In this case it is possible that the coordinator assumed that the offer of the donor from the matching agency must be of the same blood type for the offer to have been made in the first place.

Alternatively: did the surgeon on call that night make the same assumption when the coordinator called and suggested that this particular donor might suit the particular recipient? Certainly it was not my practice to ask if blood types were identical if the coordinator called and stated that he/she had a donor for a specific recipient. Did these conversations take place at times of fatigue or stress on the part of any one of the people in the communication chain? All these possibilities exist, of course, and in the end, blame will be placed on a single individual if not on the system itself. Hopefully the improvements that are made will not inhibit the smooth functioning of the program.

Unfortunately, following such circumstances new regulations place added burdens on an already beleaguered program. Truly the cure is sometimes worse than the disease, wherein the administrative remedies are sufficiently cumbersome and odious as to prevent flexibility and efficiency. Nor should the public alter their opinion of the calibre of the particular program. They probably made a human error. You can be assured that they will correct it. They are not unique. Emerging technology and innovative programs will always experience the unfortunate outcome that is created from human error, systems failure, or the unexpected. The loss of the space shuttle *Columbia* is just another example within an area of emerging expertise that functions on the limits of our knowledge seeking to push the envelope further. In space travel and in surgery complications are expected. They are unfortunate but not always avoidable. We progress when we gradually reduce their incidence or their ramifications by the quality control mechanisms we establish to analyze and correct each occurrence. The challenge is to ensure that the corrective mechanisms are not an excessive reaction that places unreasonable restraints on the program development.

In this case, the end result would not be altered by the problems encountered with the donor. The dissection of the left lung became tedious and one of the most meticulous I have ever performed. The surgeons in Toronto would have a long wait for our arrival and the anaesthesia time would be greatly prolonged. However, the lungs provided were of high quality. There was minimal damage from the dissection, which in the end proved insignificant and temporary. In addition, we would later learn from the family of the donor that the tumour removed was benign and had not been in the lung but rather had arisen in the neural tissues within the chest cavity. Nonetheless, our protocol would in the future insist on a direct contact from the donor surgeon to the recipient surgeon after the lungs had been visually inspected. Until that conversation occurred, the recipient operation could not commence.

Ann survived her transplant and became the first successful recipient of a double lung graft that did not also involve the use of the donor heart. The double lung procedure designed by Alec Patterson would very quickly replace heart/lung transplantation as the procedure of choice for patients with septic lung disease such as cystic fibrosis and bronchiectasis. Although the operative technique would be improved by others over time, the basic concept of transplanting the lungs without the heart was to become accepted worldwide within a few short years. Such would ensure that the donor heart could be used for a separate patient awaiting a cardiac transplant for isolated cardiac failure. More than this, however, Ann's success firmly established isolated lung transplantation as accepted surgical practice by broadening its capacity to provide an alternative to all patients suffering from respiratory failure irrespective of the cause. For those of us in Toronto, it was the realization of the original dream. Tom Hall had established feasibility. Ann Harrison brought to the program a sense of maturity and a confidence that the dream had substance.

The magnitude of Ann's personal contributions to the program and to transplantation in general had not been anticipated. Even before Tom's death in 1990, she had begun to assume the role of spokesperson for the recipients, both potential and transplanted. She became an advocate for the Toronto program and a symbol of the success of transplantation in general, speaking to hospitals, organizations, and governmental agencies. Her energy and dedication to the cause of patients with respiratory difficulties achieved more recognition for pulmonary transplantation than any advocacy by physicians themselves. She embodied in her enthusiasm and obvious functional success all that the program was about. Her sincerity could never be doubted. At great length she discussed with the ICU staff her perceptions of how it felt to be a recovering patient in an intimidating environment. In so doing, she shed new light on the psychological aspects of the post-operative period— insights that were to reshape our thinking and eventual practice.

Ten years after her transplant, Ann arrived unannounced in my office after she had undergone a

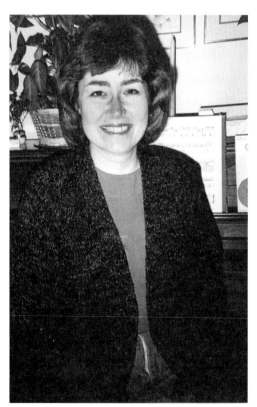

Figure 11. Ann Harrison.

surveillance bronchoscopy by one of our respirology colleagues. Bronchoscopy had become a routine aspect of rejection monitoring. Performed under local anesthesia, it involved the biopsy of several areas of the transplanted lung. A small (I'm sure it appears not so small to patients) fibre optic scope is inserted either through the mouth or nose and advanced down into the trachea. The lining of the trachea is no less sensitive than the throat itself and thus there is always a variable amount of coughing and gagging until the local anesthetic takes hold. If you can recall the sensation of aspirating food or water while eating you will be close to appreciating the experience. A series of tiny biopsies can be taken deep in the lung through the instrument. The biopsies were then scrutinized for the microscopic appearance of rejection. Thus it had become possible to diagnose rejection even if the patient was not yet symptomatic and the x-rays were still normal. It was reasoned that augmented immunosuppression at such a point when the patient remained asymptomatic would stand a greater chance of successfully repressing the rejection process. It had become an established practice to perform bronchoscopy at routine intervals following a transplant.

At her tenth anniversary, Ann questioned the requirement of undergoing the procedure when in actual fact it had not produced any signs of rejection in her case for several years. She found the entire procedure not only uncomfortable but also a source of considerable anxiety. Several years after that visit, her question would be officially answered in the medical literature. Indeed, the requirements for interval bronchoscopy would be significantly altered, much as she had predicted.

I do remember our conversation at the time. I had attempted to justify the ongoing application of the procedure in her case simply because she was the longest surviving transplant recipient. I reasoned that each new biopsy might yield novel information. She responded with a knowing smile that she could accept this opinion as long as the procedure could be performed under general anesthesia and by myself. Given her contributions to the program, this was a hard request to discount. The danger, however, lay in the fact that other recipients could make a similar request. But this was Ann and our relationship by this time was such that refusal was impossible. I granted her request, and in so doing acquired the wrath of the pulmonologist directing the program at that time. Establishing such a precedent was an inappropriate action on my part, but I have never regretted the response. It seemed that Ann had bought for herself a position of privilege. As it turned out, she was correct in questioning the frequency of the procedure and the protocols were substantially altered.

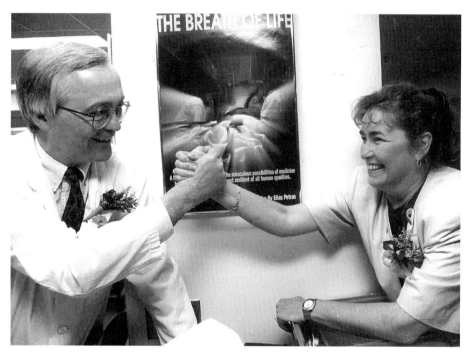

Figure 12. Ann Harrison and the author, *Toronto Star*, 1996.

Ann died in 2001 from a cerebral hemorrhage unrelated to her transplant. Several years before her death, she and I participated in a celebration of the success of multi-organ transplantation at the Toronto General Hospital. It was a media event designed to promote donor awareness, and as a result our picture together appeared on the front page of one of the Toronto newspapers (Figure 12). I have a copy hanging on the wall of my office. It serves to remind me of this wonderful woman and of the contributions that patients themselves make to the progress of medicine. After all, patients are the focus of all we undertake. Ann was the ultimate patient. Every time I see the picture I recall that stormy night in Kingston so many years ago. How easily the result could have been otherwise. How tenuous is our hold on success!

The defining feature of donor management was the unique social and/or clinical situation that surrounded each case. Certainly there were those that were routine, where everything just seemed to fall into place. There were many where I was just too tired to remember or even appreciate the black comedy that accompanied my own clinical activity. I recall short segments but the rest is so blurred in time that the accuracy of the detail is suspect.

However, I do recall one trip to Thunder Bay, Ontario, at the end of a particularly long week. I was so tired that I was not only sound asleep throughout the plane trip but had to be awakened by the resident when the cab arrived at the hospital in Thunder Bay. It was 0300 hours and I remained in a fog for some time thereafter. The recall is poignant for me because I remember at one point the resident asking me if I really wanted to cut the structure that my actions suggested I was definitely preparing to do. The structure was a significant branch of the pulmonary artery. I am thankful that he was not inhibited from commenting, for such an action on my part would have led to a major disaster from which we might not have recovered.

This was the first time that I began to appreciate the debate in the lay press and in the medical journals concerning fatigue amongst medical residents. There had been articles published suggesting that the judgment of the residents was adversely affected after twenty-four hours on call. Like most surgeons of my generation, I defended the rigourous training programs wherein young trainees are expected to function at a high level of competence in decision making roles for periods of twenty-four to forty-eight hours with little respite and at times with only snatches of sleep. The experience generated by being available for long periods of time seemed especially important. There was also the argument that once in practice, the surgeon would be expected to perform with little rest at all hours of the day and night by virtue of physician shortages and obligations to patients within the practice. Certainly the latter is true, but it is also clear that there are indeed limits on the ability to function at the appropriate level when fatigue is prominent.

I had realized that limit in Thunder Bay that night and was embarrassed by the incident. Most important, it was apparent that I was unaware of my own limitations at the time. The same fatigue that impaired my technical performance could also seriously affect my judgment. This was in 1997, twenty years into my independent practice of surgery; I have to wonder how often in previous years there were more subtle instances where either technical skill or judgment was less than optimal—sufficiently subtle that it went unrecognized.

There are several other donor episodes that remain firmly entrenched in memory either because I took notes at the time or indeed they were oft repeated to whoever would listen to the details. There are two worth mentioning here.

The first involved a daytime trip to Oshawa. The city is located outside Toronto and is approximately a one-hour drive. There was some debate during the planning for the donor run as to whether we would travel by ambulance, limousine, or helicopter. The reason for the discussion focused on Toronto's rush hour. Getting to Oshawa during the day would not be a problem, especially as the trip there was not the critical piece of the puzzle. It would be the predictability of the *return trip* that created concern. Although ambulances can manage reasonably well in traffic with the sirens and lights, there is no doubt that even their progress through the height of rush hour can be problematic. Thus, considering the time factor, the helicopter was unquestionably the best option. This was in the mid-nineties, a time of cost restraint in health care across the country. Of our options, the helicopter might be the most desirable and convenient means of transport for the team, but was certainly the most expensive. Given the relatively short distance, that option was quickly eliminated. A limousine would be fine on the outbound trip but the absence of a siren and a driver accustomed to traffic violations would greatly impair our return trip. Thus, for the return trip we settled upon an ambulance. This seemed reasonable, as we would be returning to the city when the traffic should be largely going in the opposite direction at the end of the workday.

I made the trip with Ziv Gamliel, one of my residents at the time, accompanied by Chris Freitag, one of our MORE coordinators. The outbound trip was uneventful given the fact that we were not in a hurry. I do recall that we huddled in the back of the limousine in our lab coats and OR greens. Since it was a short trip, there was no reason to change into street clothes just to do the same thing when we arrived in Oshawa.

The extraction of the lungs proceeded without event. We were somewhat delayed waiting for the liver team to arrive, but once we started the case, no particular problems were encountered. As was our custom, I asked Chris to notify the ambulance service of our imminent departure just as I was beginning the infusion of the cold preservative solution into the pulmonary artery. We generally projected about forty-five minutes from that point. The recipient case was already well underway in Toronto, as they anticipated a rather quick return from such a short distance. We were looking forward to a very short ischemic time.

At the same time, Ziv broached the ever-important subject of food. Attempting to sandwich in time for eating is a constant concern of surgical residents and transplant surgeons. You never know when the next opportunity may arise. We had already missed lunch and with the prospect of involvement with the recipient looming as a reality upon our arrival in Toronto, this suddenly acquired priority status. I had noticed a Pizza-Pizza shop shortly after we had exited from the 401 highway. Thus I suggested to Chris that after speaking with the ambulance dispatch he should order a large pizza that we would pick up as we left the city. We would have ample time to consume it en route to Toronto. "Add several cokes," Ziv interjected.

The problems began when we arrived at the emergency entrance, lungs in tow, only to find that there was no ambulance. It could be we had been faster than usual, but I recall Chris responding to my query in that regard that indeed we were about right on time. It was now after 1600 hours, and rush hour would soon be in full swing.

"So where are they, Chris?" I answered caustically.

Chris was always calm and cool. "Don't worry, they'll be here in a minute," he replied. Ten minutes later, I was pacing up and down the ambulance ramp in my greens and lab coat mumbling various threats and punishments for the ambulance attendants. This prompted Chris to dial up the ambulance dispatch service on his cell phone to request an update on their arrival. He was informed that they had left for the hospital twenty minutes previously.

"See if they can at least call them and find out where the hell they are, Chris." I was losing patience. I had very little left to lose at this point.

He called. They were on their way. No further clarification was forthcoming. At 1645 hours I was beyond myself with agitation. I had spoken to the OR in Toronto and indeed they were ready for me. They were doing nothing. The patient was asleep, chest opened, and the surgeons were in the lounge, leaving the resident to stand by scrubbed in the OR. Rush hour was upon us. Our trip was now expanded to at least an hour and half and perhaps two hours. Just as my vindictive comments approached new heights, an ambulance slowly rolled up the ramp.

"You the guys going to Toronto General?" queried the attendant as he opened the passenger door.

"No—we're doctors standing out here in our greens to escape our responsibilities inside. Where have you guys been?" I rather ungraciously responded.

"Oh we had to go for gas," replied the driver casually as he came around the front of the ambulance.

"Well we've been waiting for you for forty-five minutes. Just get back in and let's go," Chris said.

Totally nonplussed, he responded, "So we're in a hurry? You want a quick trip with sirens and lights?"

"No question. Just move it," said Chris.

These guys were unbelievable. Not a word of apology or concern. I decided at that point further comment was unlikely to be constructive or understood and just climbed into the back of the ambulance with Ziv and Chris.

As we sped away from the hospital, I spoke with the team in Toronto on the cellular hook up and informed them that we would keep in touch as far as the traffic was concerned and its effect on our arrival time. The surgeon in charge of the recipient wanted to discuss a complication that had occurred in one of the patients we had transplanted the previous week. The conversation was further prolonged about other aspects of our practice. Sitting on the bench across from me in the back of the ambulance, Ziv was obviously concerned about something. Finally he interrupted.

"Ah, Dr. Todd, let's not forget the pizza."

I could barely hear him above the ambulance siren and the other surgeon occupying my one ear. Chris, however, was aware of my hearing difficulties.

"We have to stop for the Pizza, Tom," said Chris.

"Oh, right—are we close?" I questioned as the ambulance swung hard to the left as it sped through a red light. "Tell the guy driving to stop at Pizza-Pizza, will you?"

There followed the rather incongruous sight of a speeding ambulance with lights flashing pulling up abruptly in front of

Pizza-Pizza just after running a red light. This was followed by Ziv hopping out the back doors garbed in his greens and lab coat. Running into the shop with funds in hand he emerged quickly with the pizza and drinks. In moments we were underway once again, passing several cars for the second time as we loudly meandered in and out of traffic. Subsequently, I did have to apologize to the driver for my criticism of his tardy arrival and for emphasizing the need for speed only to have him stop for our repast in the midst of his wild run.

We arrived in Toronto somewhat late, as anticipated, but the ambulance driver was actually rather good and managed to create many interesting diversions within the traffic. The resultant swinging and swaying in the back of the vehicle did manage to plant some of the pizza sauce on our lab coats, and we arrived in Toronto looking more like pizza chefs than surgeons. Nonetheless, the surgery went smoothly and the patient did well, aided no doubt by the satiety of the surgical staff.

The other episode that remains fresh in my mind occurred early on in our distant retrieval experience. I no longer recall the intended recipient, but do recall that the offer came from Sudbury in Northern Ontario on a day when winter came to call with a vengeance. The donor seemed perfect. We were well into our planning for the procedure when we received word that the international airport was closed due to the winter storm that was affecting most of the province. The MORE program assured us that Sudbury would do their best to maintain the donor in the hopes that by the next day the storm would permit travel.

It was a significant storm. I have never been one to shy from the roadways when snow and ice perform their destructive rituals at the end of winter. Yet on this occasion, I decided to leave my car at the hospital and manage my way home on the subway and bus system when the day came to an end. The authorities had warned motorists to stay off all the highways and city roads if possible. The subway station looked like New York's Times Square at New Year's, despite the fact that it was by this time seven o'clock in the evening. It appeared as if everyone else had come to the same conclusion and had delayed their normal departure time to avoid the crowds and confusion that were unfortunately still present. It took a long time to find room on a subway car and I was by this time annoyed at my reticence to drive. There was still only standing room when the train approached the Old Mill station accompanied by my pager blaring away on my belt. The digital read-out contained the coordinator's number at the hospital. I had yet to purchase a cell phone and thus exited the car at the Old Mill station to find a pay phone.

"Dr. Todd, we have found a plane that can leave from the Island airport tonight. Sudbury will open their airport for the donor flights," said the voice on the other end of the line.

"I'm already in the west end; do we have to leave from the Island? Can't we go from Pearson?" I queried in response. The Island airport is a small local traffic airport situated on Toronto Island. The Island sits in the bay at the foot of the city streets. Pearson is the international facility located in the west end near my home.

"No, Pearson is still closed but they'll take you from the Island," she replied. The thought of the international airport closed while the local airport had reopened was not a confidence-inspiring scenario for someone who is an anxious flyer in the first place.

"You sure this is okay?"

"Yeah, they say no problem, but we have to hurry, as the Island may have to shut down again if the snow continues." Another reassuring comment! "We knew you had left the hospital, so Dr. Cooper said to send the police out to your home to pick you up."

"There's a problem—I got your page on the subway. I'm at the Old Mill station." It briefly occurred to me that perhaps I was still going to avoid this.

"No problem—I'll call them and Dispatch will just reroute them directly to you there. I'll tell them you'll meet them outside the station—okay?"

I strode off to the exit with visions of an aircraft bumping along through the worst storm of the year with the airsickness bag clutched tightly in my fist, not quite grateful that Joel had volunteered me for this task. Easy for him to make the decision; *he* didn't have to take this trip! I recalled one of his own favourite phrases when commenting on the willingness of internists to recommend surgery for high-risk patients: The Courage of the Non-combatant. I sure felt like the combatant, quite ready to throttle the non-combatant. I heard the police sirens within a few minutes of walking to the street from the subway station. These guys continued to amaze me. We headed directly to the ferry that connects to the Island across the western gap with the mainland—a narrow waterway through which pleasure craft access Lake Ontario from the safety of the harbour. The officer explained that its normal hours of operation had ceased about fifteen minutes earlier but that they were waiting for us. The MORE coordinator and my resident were already there.

The resident that night was David Sugarbaker, currently the head of Thoracic Surgery at the Peter Bent Brigham Hospital in Boston. Exiting the ferry on the island, we realized that we would have to walk through the unplowed roadway to the terminal. Having arrived at work that day without boots only added to the unpleasantness. However, such annoyances were quickly minimized by the vision of our intended aircraft.

No streamlined jet waited us on the tarmac. Rather we were assigned a double-prop cargo plane, apparently the only one granted clearance for such a trip. Our accommodation was cold and sparse. We had jump seats—no comfort spared. If there was heat in the portion of the plane accommodating us, it was not apparent. The coordinator had, however, arranged for the ubiquitous pizza. By the time we were airborne and the pizza displayed on a crate between us it was hard to determine if this was an uncooked frozen pizza or actually had come from an oven at some point. Nonetheless, the actual trip to Sudbury was, if not smooth, certainly not as frightening as I had anticipated.

We arrived calm. However the pilots informed us as we taxied to the terminal that the roads were sufficiently snowbound as to preclude even ambulance traffic. Thus they had arranged for helicopter transport to the roof of the hospital. The chopper had already taken the Ottawa heart team to the hospital, as their plane had arrived ahead of ours, and we would need to wait in our aircraft until it returned. It was at least warmer on the ground than it had been in flight.

Once we arrived at the hospital, the surgical side of things proceeded without event. We had an excellent working relationship with the Ottawa group. In the change room before entering the operating room, my own team discussed the problems we might have with ischemic times, given our varied modes of transportation and the continuing storm. This would be exaggerated by the fact that the heart would be removed first and they would leave with the helicopter ahead of us. Our wait on the tarmac for the chopper's arrival had seemed overly long upon our arrival. Given that there would be no more than fifteen minutes between their readiness for departure and ours, a further significant delay seemed possible.

We also recognized that their ischemic time was not as critical as ours. Thus it was that we behaved badly. The briefcase of the cardiac surgeon was obvious by virtue of the initials on the handle. We shared the change room but they were already in the operating room. It became rather simple to have the briefcase travel to another area in the locker room and to find its way under one of the benches that was conveniently covered with dirty scrubs. Their departure would be unavoidably delayed in the search for the briefcase. It seemed a great idea at the time.

We completed the removal of the lungs in record time and hurriedly assembled all our instruments. Having literally run down the corridor to the locker room, we not unexpectedly found the heart team frantically searching for the missing briefcase. The helicopter was at the roof, waiting. Wishing to be constructive and in an attempt to assuage our guilt, we did suggest that perhaps the cleaning staff had moved it. Did they check at the nursing station or in the surgeon's lounge? We changed quickly and as we were leaving deigned to assist them in their search. One of us spotted the briefcase under a bench, hidden by carelessly flung scrubs. Conveniently, this happened as one of our members was already at the elevator for access to the roof. As they were not yet ready, it seemed only appropriate that we head off first to the airport, especially as our ischemic time was the more critical. Their graciousness in accepting this solution prevented any light commentary on the trip back to the airport. We were pleased with the outcome but hardly proud of ourselves.

Our return trip to Toronto was a repeat of the inbound. However, as we landed at the Island airport, we were informed that as it was now about three o'clock in the morning, the ferry was definitely not available. Instead, we would be taken across the harbour in a police boat. Unfortunately, the police boat would be at a dock accessible only through deep, drifting snow. Retribution for our sins, I thought as I struggled through the knee-deep snow in my dress pants and loafers.

Our actions were further rewarded when we recognized that the police dock was not at the narrow Western gap but rather situated across from the city at some considerable distance. The police boat was not enclosed. The harbour was choppy. As a result, our appearance once we arrived at the mainland was not respectable.

There followed a ride to the hospital in a police van. I was to remain chilled for several days, even though the transplant itself was a great success. We had managed to secure another donor. To do so, we had travelled by a speeding police car, a ferryboat, cargo plane, helicopter, police boat, and a police van, interspersed with two expeditions through knee-deep snow in city clothes. We had in addition acted deviously and inappropriately with our medical compatriots. It was a long night and I slept soundly on the subway riding home the next evening after another day at the hospital. This time I was simply too tired to drive. I do, however, recall David Sugarbaker's exclamation when we trundled down into the police boat: "Man, has this been great! The only thing we haven't travelled by is dogsled!"

CHAPTER 9

Departures and Returns

In the late 1980s, we basked in our success. Isolated lung transplantations—both single and double lung—were firmly entrenched as feasible solutions to respiratory failure. Toronto was the recognized world authority. We organized seminars that attracted registrants from around the world. Pulmonary programs in other university centres were anxious to initiate their own programs. Joel, Alec, and I were invited to speak at conferences with an ever-increasing frequency. International invitations to attend universities and conferences were common occurrences. Thoracic trainees throughout North America competed for our residency and research positions. Research fellows from European and Asian programs came to spend one to three years working in the transplant laboratory. We were on the pinnacle of academic thoracic surgery with no apparent end in sight.

It was true that Griff Pearson, by virtue of his innovative surgical skill and his dynamic personality, had already positioned us securely in the forefront of international regard. However, lung transplantation had become the holy grail of thoracic surgery. It had eluded the best thoracic surgeons for over twenty years. For our group, it had provided the final push to the thoracic surgical summit. But it was not to last.

It was not long before the invitations to speak at meetings and universities evolved into seductive recruitment ventures. Most of them involved academic promotion, and those in the USA provided a significant economic advantage. I had been asked to the Mayo Clinic in late 1987. I was overwhelmed with their resource base and work ethic. The opportunity to be innovative was apparent in their attitude and no-nonsense approach. Unlike in Canada, the thinking of physicians and the administration appeared to be harmonious. The physicians wanted to increase volume and provide superior patient care. The same was true for the administration. Both were undoubtedly driven to some extent by profit motives, in that the greater the volume the larger the profit for both parties, given that medical care in that jurisdiction was a business. Nonetheless, quality of patient care and the comprehensiveness of its availability were also issues for both.

The skeptics amongst you will no doubt think otherwise, and for some physicians the cynicism is appropriate. But for the majority I contend that quality was just as important. For example, while being interviewed at the Mayo by a senior member of the administrative staff, I was asked if it would be my intention to seek involvement of the Clinic in a major thoracic clinical trials group with which Toronto had substantial participation. After I responded affirmatively, the administrator noted that the studies currently underway required the completion of additional CT scans in patients with lung cancer, scans that were not actually indicated for the clinical care but were for research. Having dealt with Canadian hospital administrations, I anticipated that I had just placed any hopes of a firm job offer in jeopardy. On the contrary, however, the fellow was pleased with my response and went on to comment that they would consider adding another CT scanner to the list of requests that I had already suggested. This was support of research, hardly an opportunity for the Mayo Clinic to make further profit. However, as promising as the opportunity might have been, I declined.

Basically, the attractions offered by other institutions were appealing. Thus the fact that one of our group was about to leave the fold should not have been met with surprise. In retrospect, it was more a case of who would go first. Nonetheless, I had naively assumed that we were all to remain in Toronto. It was akin to relishing the old days of hockey wherein a team tended to remain intact for years on end and premium players could remain on the roster indefinitely. It should have been readily apparent that the group could not remain intact. Any one of us was in a position to assume a leadership role and there was only room for one such in Toronto. The pattern had been seen in other world-class units over the years. In fact, medicine is indeed much like a modern championship sports team. After a few years it breaks apart. First one leaves. For the others, it is never the same, and one by one the diaspora occurs. With Joel at the helm of Thoracic Surgery, Griff Pearson as the chief of the Department of Surgery at TGH, and Bob Ginsberg the chief of Surgery at the Mt. Sinai hospital across the street, it certainly appeared as if Alex Patterson and I would be the ones to move on to leadership positions elsewhere. But there was still surprise awaiting us all.

At a Thoracic meeting in Texas in 1988, I met Joel one morning for breakfast at his request. We met at one of those ubiquitous little coffee bars tucked away in the corner of the convention centre. He had been to San Diego, ostensibly to speak at the university, and had arrived a day or two late for the Dallas meeting.

Our schedules in and out of Toronto had been frantic. We had recently shared very little private time together despite the fact that our offices were side by side on the tenth floor of the hospital. I always enjoyed the academic and social banter that we shared. He was and always has been a stimulating fellow, and I believe that we both enjoyed the flow of ideas that usually accompanied one of our conversations. In addition, we shared a strong religious background, albeit within entirely different religious faiths. Joel's father was a Rabbi and my father had been a Christian Minister. We both possessed an intensive if not encyclopedic knowledge of Hebrew history and of comparative religions. I believe that I learned more about Christianity from my Jewish friend and partner than I ever did from discussions with my Christian acquaintances. Whether medical or religious in nature, conversations with Joel Cooper were something to relish.

That morning I really didn't notice that he was not his animated and argumentative self. Nor did I pick up the significance of his comment that he had stopped at Washington University in St. Louis on his way back from San Diego. I recall that the true purpose of our early morning meeting did not penetrate my unobservant self until he told me that he had some time before determined that thirteen years was more than enough time to spend in one academic centre. As he had been in Toronto since 1972, the reality of our conversation began to edge its way into my consciousness. After that prelude, it was then not a real surprise when he informed me that he had been to San Diego to look at a position there. Word travels fast and before he left San Diego he had received a call from St. Louis inviting him to stop there en route to Dallas. St. Louis had never been a consideration, he explained, but after his visit it appeared as if indeed this was the place he had been looking for.

Basically, he told me that morning that he thought he would leave Toronto by the spring. This was enormous news with significant ramifications. Joel had been a permanent fixture! The transplant program was his child. The move just did not seem to make sense. From a professional standpoint, it appeared like a lateral move. He was already chief of the Service in Toronto. Although the Thoracic division in St. Louis had a notable history, the Toronto Thoracic group was recognized worldwide for its innovation and academic record.

Joel himself provided the answers. He foresaw the decline in Canadian academic medicine that would occur throughout the next decade (and unfortunately beyond). He was determined to avoid the frustrations attendant upon the lack of front-line technology, ever-increasing surgical waiting lists, and disappearing dollars directed towards innovative clinical and basic science research. He was also clear on one other point. The level of remuneration in Canada was not commensurate with the work ethic that characterized the Toronto General in those years. With four children headed for higher education at the best schools in the continent, he would be unable to provide them with the access they academically deserved. Ten years later, I was to realize that Joel's predictions were accurate. By that time, our resource base for the program had decreased substantially. Waiting lists for elective surgery, including those for cancer, had quadrupled. I was working even longer hours and my effective income had fallen about thirty percent. Newer technology was slow in coming, if ever.

I left our early morning meeting with apprehension but also considerable anticipation. Joel was one of a team of seven surgeons that included myself. Surely everything we had built could survive his departure unscathed. On the other hand, I suspected he was at least partially correct in his assessments. Time and circumstance were about to bring significant change. I was forty-three years of age and felt like a schoolboy about to change grades—one of my teachers and mentors, the founder of our program, would shortly no longer be a part of my everyday life.

We had assumed that Bob Ginsberg would take over as the Division chief, as he already had acquired administrative experience and was well known in international thoracic circles. Indeed, he was offered the position. The recruitment of a new leader is usually an opportunity to acquire added resources through the process of negotiation. By 1989, we were in significant need, as the restrictions on spending and the debts of the Ontario hospitals had quickly led to deficiencies. As a division, we discussed the areas that Bob would address in his negotiations. The list was modest compared to what one might expect to see demanded by a prospective appointee in the USA or indeed in Canada prior to that era of fiscal restraint.

The Toronto General and the Toronto Western hospitals had undergone what would prove to be the first of several hospital mergers across the country. Our division had been vocally critical of the undertaking and as a result we were not popular with the administration. Nonetheless, it came as a surprise when we heard from Bob that the hospital had rejected most of his requests. We were astonished. At first I speculated that Bob must have had an extensive list of personal demands. Our list of required equipment seemed so basic that I presumed the hospital would see the logic irrespective of Bob's pending appointment. Certainly the equipment was considered a prerequisite for us to continue to permit the expected expansion of the transplant program. We were about to learn what Joel had already understood. Excellence and world-class achievement would stand for little with the advent of cost containment.

Shortly thereafter, Bob announced that he would accept the position of head of Thoracic Surgery at the prestigious Memorial Sloan Kettering Cancer Center in New York. Another link in the chain had broken, and the polish on the brass seemed dull and tarnished. For Bob, the move was to provide him with a resource base and level of support that would vault him into international pre-eminence in cancer treatment and research. He became a surgical star. He would return to Toronto more than ten years later to replace me as division head of thoracic surgery at a time when the division's need was desperate. Unfortunately for us all, he would succumb to lung cancer in 2003. Despite his role as a thoracic surgeon, he had continued his smoking habit.

Within six months, I accepted the position of chief of surgery at the Ottawa Civic Hospital and by April 1990 had departed Toronto. Although appointed as the head of surgery at the Civic, my real interest in the position related to transplantation. At the time the cardiac transplantation program in Ottawa was probably the most successful and well organized in the country. There was a small kidney program at the Ottawa General, the other teaching hospital for the University of Ottawa, but otherwise there was no other transplant activity in Ottawa. The addition of lung transplantation would greatly complement the cardiac program and hopefully provide the focus for the development of a full-scale, multi-disciplinary transplant program for the university.

That was certainly the vision of the departmental chairman at the university, who fortunately was also the director of cardiac surgery as well as being a senator in the national government. His influence was extensive, and I was persuaded that the opportunities for growth were significant. It seemed a logical move. I would obtain a more influential position that would provide the administrative base for the institution of a full-scale program in organ transplantation. In addition, the vice-president of research and administration had unfortunately acquired pulmonary fibrosis and would require a lung transplant in the not too distant future. As a result, the commitment of the Civic hospital to the entire idea of transplantation was solid. It all seemed logical—it was time to leave Toronto.

But the departures were not yet complete. Two years later, Alex Patterson left to join Joel in St. Louis. Mel Goldberg left to direct thoracic surgery at the Fox Chase Cancer Institute in Philadelphia. By 1993, of the original seven surgeons only Griff Pearson and Tim Winton, the latter our junior partner in 1989, were left.

Success in Ottawa seemed, as I noted above, just a matter of time. There were, however, two other factors in the equation, one I should have appreciated and the other quite unexpected. With regards to the former, I quickly learned that the University of Ottawa is a microcosm of the linguistic and cultural divisions in Canada. It is a fully bilingual University—an admirable achievement. However, this singular attribute provided for its undoing in the Medical Faculty. There are two teaching hospitals that were irrevocably separated at that time along linguistic lines. The normal competitiveness that exists between academic institutions was thus magnified. It became apparent that there was marginal hope in succeeding with the development of a program in one hospital without the other's providing political obstacles that were not so subtly veiled as being of medical import.

A prime example was provided to me during an unrelated meeting organized by the Dean of Medicine as he was attempting to structure a more formal relationship with the Faculty of Medical Arts and Science. The latter oversees the education of nurses, physiotherapists, and other paramedical disciplines. I received an invitation to a strategic planning session at the faculty club that would be chaired by an outside third party, a strategic planner. As an initial part of our efforts that day, it was determined that we should establish certain principles and priorities. Our first exercise would be to determine the objective measures of academic excellence. I was about to learn more about tact and negotiation in that session than in the previous twelve years of clinical practice in Toronto.

The planner situated himself at the head of a long table of leaders from both faculties, busily scribing our suggestions on a flip-chart. Each of us in turn was to make a suggestion for our scribe to enter on the flip-chart for discussion. I loved discussion. I do recall that my first suggestion as a measure of academic excellence was the number of peer-reviewed grants received annually by the faculty. When it came to the Dean of the Faculty of Medical Arts and Science, she stated that a good measure of academic excellence was the determination of whether all courses raised issues of gender. I was surprised that no comment was made by the other participants. It did occur to me that although such was an admirable objective in terms of content, it really was not a measure of the academic excellence of the program.

I cannot recall my second suggestion, but remember thinking it was pretty good (surgical ego again). Today I wish I had been more intent on understanding the political nuances that permeated the academic air in that room. The second suggestion from the dean of the other faculty caught me completely by surprise and afforded, I thought naively, a chance to discuss the entire problem of linguistic apartheid that I had witnessed in my early months in Ottawa. She stated that a measure of academic excellence was whether all programs were delivered in both official languages.

Would I had remained quiet! But no—I had to respond. At least I was sufficiently politically sensitive to note that the attainment of omnipresent bilingualism was admirable. However, I went on to note that we should not confuse that with excellence. I noted that it would be possible to have programs and courses that were of inferior quality whether bilingual or unilingual. I stated that bilingualism itself was not the appropriate measure. Pleased with my point, I failed to appreciate that the room had become rather silent until the dean rose to her feet and provided a rather emotional litany of response in French that to this day remains incomprehensible. It may be fortunate that I understood not a word of her retort. As she sat down, I was for the first time in my life bereft of words, largely because I had no idea what she had said. A quiet voice to my right offered the following comfort: "Welcome to Ottawa."

The two hospitals were, as I have stated, divided largely along linguistic lines. Despite this, there did appear to be achievable compromise between the two factions. Sufficiently encouraged, I initiated consultations with the MORE program that would permit the entry of Ottawa into the distribution of lung donors. Indeed, a small but steady stream of referrals began to appear in my lung clinic at the Civic Hospital. The hospital had provided the resources, and I had two colleagues able and willing to provide assistance. Once MORE granted approval, I would have a number of recipients already on board to initiate the program. In Toronto, we had spent the first two years attempting to define the suitable donor. With that experience behind me, I would be able to proceed quickly once approval was granted. I was then totally blind-sided by the second factor.

The New Democratic Party of Ontario had recently been elected for the first time in the province's history. As we were poised to officially announce opening of the lung program in Ottawa, we were informed by the government that they would not permit the establishment of new transplant programs. Although the hospital had agreed to provide initial funding, further funds would simply not be provided. Driving home that night, I realized that the move to Ottawa had been a mistake and determined that it would soon be time to leave. By 1993, the position no longer offered the promise that seemed so obvious three years previously. Where to go was the question.

Toronto was interested. They had recruited two surgeons from the USA, but neither was experienced in transplantation, nor inclined to participate in such. This left only the now not-so-junior partner (Dr. Winton) performing lung transplants. Although there were several respiratory physicians capable of providing support in the pre- and post-operative phases, a solitary physician on the surgical end was not sustainable. St. Louis had rapidly expanded all its thoracic programs, and Joel was eager to bring in another Toronto expatriate.

In early 1993, I commenced discussions with both St. Louis and Toronto. The former would have reunited me with Joel and Alec and provided me with a great opportunity to organize surgical critical care at the university hospital in St Louis. It was very tempting, and in retrospect clearly the best choice. In the end, it was to be a socially driven decision. With two children attending university in Canada and two at home, a move to the United States would have divided our family geographically. Moreover, it appeared likely that if we moved to St. Louis, the two at home would eventually attend American universities when finished with high school and thus would probably reside in the United States thereafter. The geographic separation would be indefinite.

Toronto offered the opportunity for me to be chief of Thoracic Surgery (Joel's old position) and afforded the chance to rebuild the transplant division and the training program. There was a new administration in place, suggesting that perhaps the philosophy of restraint might be over. The lure of being the head of the thoracic division previously run by Pearson and Cooper was attractive. Thus in 1993, I returned to Toronto and commenced the final chapter of my involvement in lung transplantation. Looking back, the lack of insight that I brought to the situation is staggering.

Years of financial restraint had taken their toll. I had known that things would change, and indeed they had. The thoracic operating time had been severely reduced. The number of assigned beds was about seventy-five percent of the quota we had enjoyed in the eighties. Even our old operating rooms had been given to others to be replaced by those barely large enough to accommodate our equipment and staff. All of Joel's predictions had come true. Not predicted, however, was the disharmony within the division itself. The camaraderie and interpersonal support that characterized the division in the nineteen eighties had disappeared. I naively thought that it could be restored.

Commencing my tenure as division head, I was aware of these things before accepting the position. What I had not anticipated was the continued severe budget restraints that would characterize Canadian medicine throughout the latter half of the 1990s. There was simply nowhere to move. Every year there were further reductions in operating dollars. I was anxious to expand the division's activities and restore its dynamic role in international thoracic surgery. The resources to do so were simply not to materialize.

We were able to re-establish academic productivity with the recruitment of Dr Keshavjee in 1995. Dr. Keshavjee had been a research fellow during my previous tenure in Toronto and had spent two years in London and Boston before returning to Toronto. His research training was superb and he would quickly establish an active and productive laboratory that was dedicated to issues pertinent to lung transplantation. However, the ability to grow clinically was greatly hampered by the lack of funds and would be realized only by augmented effort on the part of the surgeons, nurses, and support staff. Yet further growth was essential to meet the demands of the waiting list and to maintain our prominence internationally in transplantation.

With the departure of Dr. Patterson, the number of transplants had decreased by approximately twenty-five to thirty percent. One surgeon could simply not provide the same support to the program. The mortality on the waiting list had increased. With Dr. Keshavjee's exuberance and the presence of myself and Dr. Winton, we did achieve a steady increase in productivity until we greatly surpassed our previous best efforts. But this was all achieved at great personal sacrifice on the part of our entire staff. The number of staff had dwindled from the late 1980s, and thus to achieve similar, let alone increased productivity, stresses were bound to appear.

In 1987, our lung transplant program had the following staff members: one coordinator, two fellows in training (one surgical and one medical), and five surgeons with another as backup. By 1999, the numbers were one **shared** coordinator, an occasional medical transplant fellow, and three surgeons. This may not seem like a major decrease, but remember that in 1987 our annual transplant volume was about a quarter of what we achieved in 1999. In addition, all those transplanted in the intervening years required regular follow-up and attention. The numbers seeking the procedure had tripled, and with the success of the program it was apparent that the clinical restrictions on recipients that were imposed in 1983 could be relaxed. As a front-line program, we should have been leading the way in developing initiatives for the transplantation of high-risk individuals. The latter had always been my prime motivation. Thus it was obvious that we required expanded resources at least to the levels available in 1989. There were to be none. I was about to enter the most frustrating period of my career.

Not all our problems were economic. At my departure three years previously, I had begun to sense that the program was losing its personal touch with the patients. That was to be expected as we grew in size. However, the reduction in number of surgeons interested in transplantation meant that there was even *less* individual time for our involvement in the personal side of the program. As surgeons, we became technicians and critical care physicians. The comprehensive approach that permitted us to come to know all the patients on the waiting list required modification. There just were not enough hours in the day. Our exposure to patients prior to surgery and after their transfer from the intensive care unit became progressively less. Such is the norm in most transplant programs. The surgeons operate and manage the initial post-operative period, and the rest is managed by internists.

Toronto, however, had been different in the beginning. No doubt this was because we liked it that way, but also because there had been no one else to undertake these tasks at the time. No one had believed that we would ever be successful, and thus all aspects of the program had required our active participation in the early stages. The program had been ours in every sense of the word and we cherished it like a child.

Just as there had been a departure of the main players, so too had disappeared the comprehensive control that the surgical division had exercised. The program was under the control of others whose objectives resembled more that of a maintenance man than a person of innovation and challenge. Lack of funding and lack of drive and imagination made proper bedfellows. Which was the cause and which the effect was not possible to determine. Admittedly the maintenance was well done, but the program was not moving forward.

Thus upon my return I quickly found myself a participant with little opportunity to impact the organization and operation of the program in general. I found little support for innovation from the administration or my new colleagues in the transplant program. The Division of Thoracic Surgery provided sufficient challenge, and it was too easy at the start to leave the transplant program in the hands of others.

As the chief of Thoracic Surgery, I did have a chair at the business meetings of the program. Unfortunately, the objectives and the vision of the members had changed since the departure of Joel, Alec, and myself, leading to my perception of an increasing polarization that involved almost everyone else on one side of the table and myself sitting alone.

The general day-to-day operational issues differed little from previous days and there was really no controversy in that arena. But I soon became aware of the fact that our success had bred an air of complacency. They were resistant to novel ideas and to change. At first I presumed that it was my perception only. It seemed logical to assume that the others would be naturally resistant to the suggestions of a former member of the program who had abandoned them three years before. Yet as time passed it was apparent that protection of the status quo was of paramount consideration. There was a real fear of embarking on any policy or procedure that might lead to failure. There was an apparent concern that a change in our mortality or complication rates resulting from some novel idea might reflect adversely on the program as a whole. This philosophy seemed pervasive despite the fact that there was every reason to believe that attacking new frontiers might just as well result in an expansion of the program or improved delivery of the service to a larger population of patients with respiratory failure. Having been involved with the program at a time of constant change and adjustment, of daily risk-taking, where every possibility was explored, it was clear that a significant philosophical difference existed between myself and the others. Some controversial times awaited me.

CHAPTER 10

Controversies

In 1994, it was obvious that the program needed to be revitalized. I am sure there are those who would disagree, but to me it had lost its sense of adventure. It no longer looked beyond what it had achieved to determine what might be possible. To be fair, the program was involved in research protocols that were designed to evaluate novel means of immunosuppression in the post-transplant period. These were important endeavours designed to improve the long-term survival of those who survived the procedure itself. On the other hand, such did nothing to improve access to transplantation for those patients who were still denied a place on the recipient waiting list. This was in part secondary to concern that a softening of the rigid acceptance criteria would result in an increase in operative risk. Perhaps some examples will explain the situation.

Patients over the age of sixty-five were not accepted for assessment. Tom Hall was fifty-nine at the time of his transplant. Back in 1984 an arbitrary age limitation of sixty was deemed appropriate following his success. He was the oldest patient we had assessed, and so the limit was quite serendipitous. Indeed, over the succeeding ten years we had (again arbitrarily) increased the limit by five years to bring us to the magic number of sixty-five. Originally a limitation was designed to avoid a series of failures that would have, at that early stage in our development, jeopardized the program. By 1994 the program was well established and the refusal to even evaluate patients because of an arbitrary age limit was anathema to me. True, our program suffered from a lack of resources and the evaluation of this cohort would only increase the already back-breaking load. Nonetheless, I argued it would also serve as further ammunition for an increase in the resource base. It was argued that I was placing the cart before the horse. There is certainly some validity to that statement when one considers the cost-cutting atmosphere of the time.

Addressing ethical principles is never easy. I found the entire process disquieting. It simply occurred to me that we were leaving behind the opportunity to continue to advance the envelope. Although I was clearly in favour of accepting new challenges, I also recognized that there were limitations we had to accept. Our disagreements came in their definition. I disliked arbitrary rules, recognizing that every patient is different. Not all sixty-five-year-old patients are *biologically* sixty-five years old. Some would not withstand a haircut, much less a lung transplant—but the same could be said of many at age fifty-five. It wasn't age that should preclude assessment but rather the overall status of the patient, which could only be determined by the assessment itself—the process that they were denied. To predetermine the outcome was to deny the opportunity to some who might benefit, because we presume that those over sixty-five would definitely present an augmented risk. But the ethical dilemma becomes more complex when there is a shortage of donors. It was argued that it seemed appropriate to provide the scarce donor to younger folks on the waiting list who could look forward to longer years of benefit.

Age limitation was visible to the public, whereas some of the other restrictions we will note were less so. Thus it became a civil rights issue, and this limitation was the first to fall. A sixty-six-year-old man with terminal lung disease was greatly distraught when he was informed after referral by his physician that he was too old for consideration. There had been many before him denied access, but this fellow refused to simply walk out the door and accept the dictum. He threatened a civil action against the hospital and the directors of the program, accusing us of age discrimination. The hospital wanted none of the media attention this would foster, and the program was simply told to withdraw any age limits. The patient was accepted into the program. He died a few days following his transplant amid loud cries of "foul!" from some members of the program. Nonetheless, within a year I performed a successful transplant on a sixty-nine-year-old man and the entire controversy disappeared with only a low-volume groan.

But age was not the only determinant of rejection. Those who had significant co-morbidities were frequently rejected. A co-morbidity refers to an additional disease entity that might complicate the outcome. For example, a patient with concomitant coronary artery disease or associated liver or renal failure would have had difficulty gaining the approval of the assessment team. It was basically a matter of relative risk. In addition, those patients with respiratory failure sufficiently severe as to result in a requirement for ventilation were never considered appropriate. We continued with this policy despite the fact that anecdotal reports of success in the transplantation of patients on mechanical ventilators had been noted from other centres. The reluctance to undertake a transplant in a ventilated patient extended even to those individuals who had been accepted into our program prior to their deterioration and requirement for mechanical respirators. The development of ventilatory dependency automatically resulted in the patient's removal from the waiting list.

I noted that patients predisposed to a heart attack due to coronary atherosclerosis were automatically excluded. Such patients would be prone to a major cardiac event either during or after the procedure. Shortly following his arrival, Dr Keshavjee championed the idea of performing coronary artery bypass surgery at the time of lung transplantation. There had been several cases over the years where the presence of coronary artery disease had been the single factor precluding acceptance into the program. Keshavjee's argument had merit. We would already be in the chest. At least a quarter of our patients required cardio-pulmonary bypass for the transplant. So why not fix the heart at the same time? This seemed quite logical to me. However, there is no doubt that the risk of such a procedure is greater than a transplant done in isolation. Predictably, there was considerable resistance to this proposal. The objections persisted for some time. In fact, the concern was maintained even after the program agreed to accept patients with coexistent liver failure. These latter patients would undergo a combined liver and lung transplant, a procedure that in the minds of many of us carried a much greater risk. Eventually reason held forth and coronary artery disease by itself no longer constituted a reason to reject patients.

There were other groups of patients who, despite achieving the waiting list, were treated differently than the majority. One such group consisted of patients who had experienced significant rejection and required a second transplant. For this group, the procedure itself posed an augmented risk due to the operative difficulty and resultant surgical complications. A second group consisted of young patients with cystic fibrosis who were infected with an organism that was resistant to most, if not all, antibiotics. Should such an infection develop in the transplanted lungs in the early post-operative period, their demise was a certainty. A significant percentage of patients so infected and who had been transplanted to date had developed reinfection even months after a successful procedure. They were now immuno-suppressed, and, without the availability of effective antibiotics, the infection resulted in their death in a short period of time. The survival at five years of such patients was low (approximately thirty percent). Although that means seventy percent succumbed within five years following the transplant, clearly one in three did survive infection free.

In 1994, we were the only program in North America still accepting these unfortunate patients to our waiting lists. However, they and those who required a second procedure for whatever reason did not have equal access to available donors. They were placed on another list and were granted consideration only when no suitable recipient was found on the first or priority list. This practice raised ethical questions and in addition would preclude the development of experience in solving the attendant problems in these difficult patients. As long as we failed to gain experience in their management, the problems would persist. The use of marginal donors deemed inappropriate for others would increase the risks of failure. A self-fulfilling prophecy had been established.

Those supportive of the restrictions opined that it would not be fair to allocate donors to a group of patients whose chances of survival were poor. The argument had merit when one remembered that there was at least a twenty-to-twenty-five percent chance that a patient on the waiting list would succumb to his or her disease before a donor could be found. Thus it was argued we should provide the donor to those who have the best chance of survival rather than "waste" (my word) the donor organ on a high-risk case. It basically came down to how as a physician you viewed the allocation of a scarce resource. When resources, whether human or material, become scarce, a significant turmoil is created in the mind of the physician. Accepted ethical principles are called into question. You have been trained to be the protagonist of the particular patient; to be their representative. Thus you become distraught when you face the prospect that your patient may be denied life-supporting treatment; not because they are undeserving, not because there is a firm contraindication to the therapy, but rather because there is someone deemed more deserving or who has a better chance of long-term benefit. The distress becomes magnified when you are required to be the instrument that denies access to care by virtue of your participation in the donor allocation process.

The ethical dilemma is not restricted to transplantation, however. Indeed, a new ethical paradigm has arrived in medicine. The conflict is the health of the individual versus the greatest good for the greatest number. Hardly a new philosophical concept; but in medicine it has recently become of paramount concern. As resources shrink, the greatest good for the greatest number may mean very little good at all. I witnessed the initial objection of physicians to issues of dwindling resources, and experienced with considerable chagrin the response of Canadian governments both federal and provincial. The latter provides the resource in a single-payer universal system. When we would explain that we required more resource, the refrain from the financial gatekeepers was typical, with oft-repeated comments such as:

- If only the physicians would accept greater financial controls, the resources would increase.

- We need to spend more on community health and preventive medicine than on these front-line therapies that are largely unproven.

I found the latter comment particularly amusing, recognizing that if such had been the prevailing will in 1983, we would never have been permitted to spend a cent on lung transplantation— the therapy that "definitely didn't work."

But the initial objection of physicians has become muted, and the system has already begun to readjust itself. The physicians have become, if not the willing, then at times the unwitting participants in the allocation of the shrinking resource base. They make the decision as to which patient must wait nine months for an MRI scan. They are the ones who juggle the patients on long surgical waiting lists. They are the ones who must determine which of their patients with operable cancer can afford to wait the longest to access the operating room. By 1995, this was a regular occurrence in my personal practice. It occurred daily in the operating rooms across the country. Emergencies at Toronto General were classified as A, B, or C depending on acuity. Thus an "A" denoted a patient with a life-threatening situation who must be in the operating room within an hour. "B" cases had to access the room within six hours, whereas "C" cases could wait up to twenty-four hours. It was not unusual for patients with a B priority rating to wait up to ten hours and the C priorities were often lucky to pass through the sterile door of the OR suite before forty-eight or seventy-two hours. Patients with fractured hips rarely saw the operating room within the allotted twenty-four hours.

Certainly the issue of resource is important, and the cost of modern medicine is enormous. But as the physician for a patient, how do you deny care based on the fact that the chance of survival is only thirty percent, when the risk of death without therapy is one hundred percent? The patient facing death within one to two years will willingly accept a high treatment mortality in order to be provided with the opportunity of care. Tom Hall, our first transplant success, was ecstatic the night he was wheeled into the operating room with the full knowledge that no one had ever survived the procedure to leave hospital. He had been afforded his chance and his chance translated to opportunity for hundreds who followed him.

Another controversy that existed at the time of my return to Toronto involved the criteria for the acceptance of donors. Back in 1983 before the transplant on Tom Hall, we had established criteria for the acceptance of donor lungs that were based on the function of those lungs at the time of their extraction. The criteria arbitrarily set a high standard and there was a good reason for doing so. There had never been a successful transplant. Thus it seemed appropriate to ensure that the very best donor lungs were utilized in order to minimize complicating variables.

All patients and their surgeons would prefer that the donor lungs were ideal. As I have noted, we had had experience on a few occasions with lungs that were less than ideal and complications ensued. On the other hand, the obstacle to increasing the transplant rate was the paucity of donors. With fewer donors, the mortality rate on the waiting list would increase.

Prior to the departure of Dr. Patterson, the annual transplant rate had peaked at thirty-five and the operative mortality was the lowest in the world. By 1994, the annual volume had decreased to approximately twenty-four cases per year, although the results were equally impressive. The decrease in volume was multi-factorial. There had been a single surgeon, and Dr. Winton had worked himself to the point of exhaustion to maintain the quality of the program.

The number of donors available to the program had decreased for a variety of reasons. The most obvious cause was the opening of lung transplant programs in other parts of Canada. The American donors were virtually nonexistent, as programs in the United States had opened at several university centres. In several cases, these American programs were orchestrated by surgeons who had trained in our program. The success in Cleveland, Pittsburgh, Chapel Hill, and Los Angeles were in large measure secondary to the input of Toronto trainees. It became clear that the only way we were going to expand the program was to begin to accept donors whose lung function did not comply with the ideal as defined in our original criteria and to acquire another surgeon who was transplant capable. The latter was remedied by the recruitment of Dr. Keshavjee, who at that time was undertaking advanced training in France and the United States. His main focus was transplantation. He had been one of the major contributors to the transplant research program back in the late 1980s and had successfully obtained a PhD for his efforts.

The donor question, however, brought Dr. Keshavjee and me squarely into confrontation with the then program director. The thought that we might embark on a course that potentially could affect our published and enviable results was anathema to the majority of the members of the administrative committee who had managed the program after Cooper, Patterson, and I had departed for other pastures. I pointed out that the mortality rate on the waiting list had risen to over thirty percent. It seemed reasonable to assume that should the operative mortality increase, it might well be offset by a decrease in the mortality amongst the recipients desperately waiting for a chance at transplantation. The waiting patients were all on a track that led inexorably to their death within two years. I reasoned that it was better to provide them with a chance than to continue to accept such a high waiting list mortality.

Indeed, there had been publications supporting the utilization of donor lungs that did not fulfill the criteria that Joel and I had arbitrarily determined as appropriate over a cup of coffee one Sunday morning a decade before. The arrival of Dr. Keshavjee, who brought with him the original innovative spirit, greatly facilitated a shift in direction. With time, some persuasion, and simply by gradually accepting the more marginal donor without a lot of fanfare, change began to occur.

Eventually, the departure for the United States of the two internists involved in the program found us without administrative leadership. Although it created a clinical void, it also provided an opportunity for change and the creation of a renewed vision. The clinical respirology void was filled quickly by two extremely capable clinicians whom I had known for many years. Dr. Michael Hutcheon and Dr. Charles Chan accepted the challenge of joining the program. They had had very little previous exposure to transplant patients but they brought an admirable clinical expertise and the sixth sense of the experienced clinician. The quality of their work was above reproach. More importantly, they were collegial, innovative, and ready to accept new challenges. They were, however not prepared to undertake the directorship of the program. To my mind, Dr. Keshavjee represented the future of the program, but he was too young to assume this role. In addition, he had the added responsibility of directing the once-defunct research lab. The latter was blossoming under his direction, research grants were again present, and I was loath to interfere with that progress. Thus it was that the directorship of the program fell to me.

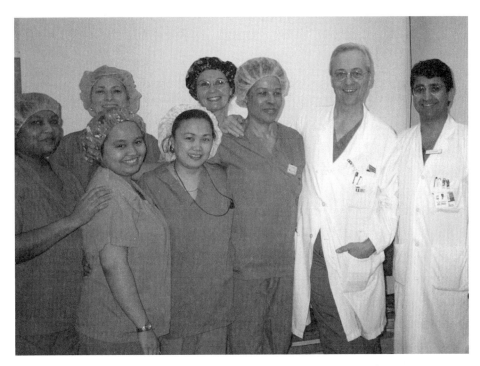

Figure 13. Dr. Shaf Keshavjee and nurses with the author, 2000.

With Dr. Keshavjee's enthusiasm, the very much appreciated collegiality of Hutcheon and Chan, and some modest change, the program assumed a new vitality. By 1999, our annual volume increased to over forty per year and the mortality on the waiting list fell to the low twenties. The research program was productive, and once again innovative publications began to appear from the Toronto program. We began to address issues that had been left without resolution for several years; issues that created ethical dilemmas for all of us to consider. We turned our attention to potentially expanding the program despite the diminishing resource base. The major issues of the ventilated patient, the re-transplant, and others excluded for reasons of co-morbidity became our focus. The debate would create animosity and anguish, but it would rejuvenate the program. We tackled the issue of the ventilated patient first.

The ability to provide mechanically generated breaths for a patient has been understood for centuries, but until the mid-twentieth century had not been employed for longer than the time required to perform an operation. Those devices that provide ventilatory support safely are the product of research and innovation carried out over the past fifty years. An entire specialty of Critical Care Medicine has been created because of the technology that has enabled us to keep patients alive for prolonged periods of time despite their inability to breathe on their own. There is no question that a multitude of patients has benefited from this development. At the same time, however, the ability to maintain patients for such protracted periods has created ethical dilemmas for the physicians and the family members—questions such as:

- When should life support be discontinued?

- Does the clinical condition carry such an ominous prognosis that life support should not even be initiated?

- Will the patient acquire sufficient functional recovery to make the effort, the pain, and the suffering worthwhile? How do we measure that?

The arrival of any new technology provides opportunities for advancement of science and medicine. However, the ramifications and possible applications of these developments may not be universally accepted, even though ostensibly they could benefit mankind. Take, for example, the advancements in the decoding of the human genome and the development of DNA technology. The potential applications are vast, but may challenge our preconceived ideas of what constitutes acceptable intervention in human and inanimate genetic structure. Cloning and the use of cells from an aborted human fetus for transplantation are prime examples. Concern with the long-term effects of genetically engineered food is another. A single advance in science is capable of creating a host of ethical questions.

Though not on the scale of these examples, the availability of lung transplantation provided us with several ethical challenges. These were to be the basis for many emotional discussions that greatly occupied the time of the transplant operations committee over the latter half of the last decade of the twentieth century. Lung transplantation was a reality. It could be accomplished with an operative mortality rate of under ten percent in appropriate patients. It was the definition of "appropriate" that created the difficulty.

Our initial forays into pulmonary transplantation had resulted in early mortality. I did not need to be reminded of those early deaths. I well knew that there had been a period of time in the early 1980s when I had thought that the program would collapse due to our inability to achieve a single success. Looking back, it became interesting to speculate on what had contributed to our ability to succeed where all others had failed. The answer to that question might well depend on the bias of the person responding and the point in time when the question was posed. In 1986, I would have responded that it was due to the several factors that we have already enumerated in this discourse in Chapters 2 and 3:

- The avoidance of steroids in the early post-operative period
- The use of omentum to revascularize the bronchial anastomosis
- The selection of patients with incipient respiratory failure but preserved nutritional status
- The avoidance of patients on ventilatory support

The ability to transplant a ventilated patient had universally proved unsuccessful until the 1990s, when anecdotal reports began to appear, highlighted by the paper from Alec Patterson and Joel Cooper in St. Louis in 2000. Certainly our experience with Jack Collins suggested that such patients were at high risk. There was also the entire history of lung transplantation that was populated with the ghosts of ventilator-dependent patients. The reasons appeared obvious. The requirement of a mechanical support of breathing benchmarks the disease as advanced and terminal unless there is an obviously reversible complication for which a short term of support is appropriate pending the latter's resolution.

Ventilated patients are largely bed bound, and this precludes exercise. Muscle strength and lean muscle mass of necessity decrease. The provision of adequate nutrition is problematic in such patients, but with modern formulations not impossible. In addition, residency in the modern ICU or indeed the hospital itself frequently leads to the contamination of the respiratory tract with highly resistant bacteria that proliferate in the face of subsequent immunosuppression. The presence of a tube through the mouth into the trachea or placed directly into the trachea (a tracheostomy) to provide the access for mechanical support ensures that these bacteria have ready access to the lung, bypassing whatever protective mechanisms exist in the upper airway. There are many reasons to suppose that the operative risk in ventilated patients is considerable.

But then the risk for any patient prior to 1983 and Tom Hall was more than considerable. It was simply put—100%. After our initial success with Tom, the question for me had not been should we transplant the ventilated patient, but rather *when and under what circumstances*. After we had established the program and had demonstrated to the doubters in the medical community that we were for real, I had begun to agitate for the start of a program that would examine the feasibility of transplanting the ventilator-dependent patient in our intensive care unit.

However, the discussion acquired less importance as the dissolution of the original team came into focus and became a reality. When I returned to Toronto General in 1993, not only had the idea languished—it was dead and buried. There was no interest in its revival. As noted, the program had assumed a complacency that cherished the success gained for it by others. It would not risk a failure. That is not to deny there were several practical and ethical problems to be addressed on this particular issue. What troubled me was the inertia blocking even discussion and consideration of our next frontier.

Joel had taught me that problems had been created for us to overcome; we merely had to work intellectually and practically by trial and error to see clearly the path to their solution. Complacency is the single greatest impediment to constructive change. The problems inherent in the transplantation of the ventilated patient are both practical and theoretical and each poses an ethical dilemma.

In addition, there loomed the very real possibility that our intensive care unit would become overwhelmed with ventilated patients in terminal respiratory failure transferred from other hospitals for the consideration of a transplant. Even I had to admit that there were practical limits to our capacity.

Compounding the discussion was the ethical concern that the allocation of the too few and precious donors to ventilated patients whose chances seemed slim indeed precluded their use for those unventilated but desperate patients on the waiting list. How did we justify such an allocation if it meant that another recipient might succumb from want of a donor?

As noted above, the same dilemma complicated the discussions surrounding two other groups of patients. First there were those whose transplant had failed due to chronic rejection— failed to the point of incipient respiratory failure once again. A second transplant we knew to be feasible. However, it was a more difficult technical undertaking with a higher operative mortality. That was not the ethical problem. The issue was simply a perception of what was fair and just. Should one individual who had already been afforded a chance preclude another from accessing his/her first opportunity at a transplant? I argued that we owed an even greater obligation to the original patient.

Granted he/she had received a donor lung and it was not a fault of the program that chronic rejection had destroyed an initially good result. Yet this patient was still our concern. He had placed his trust in us and as long as he lived we were, to my mind, contractually bound to provide whatever was feasible to save his life.

I had to agree, however, that both sides of the argument had merit. In the ideal world, we should not have been placed in the position of making choices. Irrespective of the final decision, there would be a price to pay. One group of patients would suffer for the benefit of another. Those were the realities of the moment. Unfortunately, as I write this, such choices have become commonplace in several other clinical areas throughout Canada due to the restriction of resources. It is not an ideal world. In the end, we made the decisions. Imperfect as they were, they signalled an era of development and the resurgence of risk-taking for the Toronto Program.

As far as the second group—the ventilated patients—was concerned, we agreed that those already on the recipient list who developed respiratory failure would be removed from the list. They would, however, be reassessed at frequent intervals. If there was no sign of infection and it was apparent that we would never achieve weaning, they would be considered for re-listing. This would occur rarely. To be eligible for re-listing, they would have to be stable for some time but still require the ventilator. Although this would certainly benefit several of our patients already accepted into the program, the policy would not address the critically ill, rapidly deteriorating kind of patient that Jack Collins had presented to us in 1982. It became clear that I would never win this one. The opportunity to perform a transplant in the truly desperate ventilator-dependent patient was to disappear. I would not be granted the chance to try again with the likes of a Jack Collins. But it will be done if it hasn't already. I have no doubt of that. Someone else will enjoy that success.

Re-transplantation became a reality, however. The principle

had been accepted prior to my return to Toronto, but those seeking a second transplant were placed on a separate waiting list. They were to be offered a lung only if there was no match on the main waiting list consisting of those who had never had the opportunity. It took a great deal of persuasion and some not-so-gentle cajoling, but the separate listing of these unfortunate individuals was stopped. By 1996, they assumed equal footing with the first-timers. As a result, several patients received a second chance at life. We learned much from the exercise, and it soon became an operation with comparable mortality and results. That didn't remove the concern that some first-timers might be disadvantaged. We would anguish over the decision whenever someone would die while waiting. But it worked both ways. There was a limited supply of donors. There would always be those who would lose at the allocation crap shoot. Perhaps one anecdote will suffice to justify the action.

There was a young man with cystic fibrosis who had received a transplant two years previously. His initial success was marred by rapidly progressive chronic rejection. When his lung function deteriorated sufficiently, he was considered for a second transplant. He was, however, placed on the "other list," meaning that he might be allocated a lung if it were not considered suitable for another. (Interpretation: it was not good enough for a first-timer.) He was, however, the beneficiary of the new policy and received his second chance shortly after the policy was altered. Before he left hospital after that second success, I asked him what he planned to do with such an opportunity. He smiled and said that he had always wanted to be a fishing guide and planned to do it full time in the North West Territories.

There were some members of our program who were not particularly supportive of his decision. It was considered irresponsible, as he would be too remotely located should problems develop. Our ability to monitor him closely would be impaired. But this fellow had defied the odds twice. He was not about to let another disappointment find him regretful for missing the opportunity to fulfill his lifelong dream. So he ignored the protestations of several members of the program and headed north. Three years later, I was attending a critical care conference and struck up a conversation with a respiratory physician from western Canada. He was most anxious to relate to me his encounter with our transplant patient on Great Slave Lake. While fishing, his guide asked him what he did for a living. When my colleague responded that he was a specialist in chest disease, our patient promptly removed his shirt and said, "Have I got something to show you!" Several months after that encounter, I received a letter from my patient. It recounted the same incident with the respiratory physician and then went on to detail the joy he had found with his new life. That joy was a living thing in his writing, and as I read it the decisions suddenly seemed less onerous.

The Toronto program has continued to grow. The number of annual transplants has increased to over seventy. The program thrives. I was recently at a Thoracic meeting in Toronto. Dr. Keshavjee, who has gone on to become the head of Thoracic Surgery for the University of Toronto, presented material on transplanting the unusual and difficult patient. I was thrilled to be the recipient of information that substantiated the faith I had placed in him upon his arrival at Toronto General. He and his young colleagues are recreating not only the spirit but the reality of innovation. They have performed transplants on ventilated patients and those with cancer, and have overcome technical obstacles that in 1996 we would have considered insurmountable. At one point in his presentation, he looked down at me from the podium and said, "This case will be familiar to you, Tom."

The case was of a young woman who had undergone the complete removal of one lung over ten years previously for an unusual and slow-growing cancer that can appear in multiple areas of the lung. Unlike other types of lung cancer, it spreads outside the chest only late in the disease. She had developed a recurrence in the remaining lung several years after the first operation.

At one point shortly after my return from Ottawa, she had seen Dr. Winton, seeking a transplant. The idea of transplanting such a patient with one lung already gone and the second full of cancer at that time precluded even a formal assessment. She persuaded her local physician to refer her case to me in 1999. After reviewing the case, I had to ask "Why not?" Why not try? The logistics were all within the scope of our ability. Dr. Winton objected but Dr. Keshavjee agreed. She was transplanted after my departure in 2000 for the United Arab Emirates.

This one case example reaffirmed for me that the concept of innovation, of pushing the frontiers of medicine and surgery, remains the most positive feature of medicine today. What seems impossible today will become commonplace in the future if someone merely says,

"Why not!"

CHAPTER 11

Final Departure

My transplant journal was full. The last entry contained the following.

"It's 0630 in Des Moines Iowa. The airport is quiet—at least here in the private terminal. Several cups of coffee have my brain racing although fatigue lingers in the background as sleep has escaped me for the last twenty-four hours. The first jets of the day are in the distance taxiing out to the runway surrounded by the omnipresent haze of shimmering exhaust and rippling air. Behind me I can hear the pilots being awakened unceremoniously for our return trip to Toronto. Our plane still looks cold and still in front of the terminal. But I am returning without a lung. It was simply not good enough. Another patient waits in Toronto, anxious to understand why they have been denied this donor. It's November. The morning dew on the fuselage sparkles as the sun comes up over the trees in the distance. It's a great day to be alive. There are surely great crowds of happy travellers arriving at the main terminal anticipating the start of their travel plans, and as the city of Des Moines awakens all but a few are aware that this morning has been tarnished by the death of a fifteen year old girl. I wonder if the other transplant teams are finished and if the girl's body is now empty; if brain death is now supplanted by the cessation of the heart beat. The ribald joking of the surgeons will now have been replaced by the quiet of the morning and the scurrying around of the nurses as they clean up the room. The body sits there in the midst of it all waiting to be taken to the morgue, no longer the centre of attention. It's always quiet at such times. Thinking about all that, I rejoice that the sun is still rising for me and that I can feel its heat on my face against the chill of the morning as I walk out to the waiting jet."

I had felt this special sense of life often over the past seventeen years, but on this occasion it was not to be transient. It was to be the defining moment that would alter my career and my personal life immeasurably. I had arrived in Des Moines four hours previously to extract the lungs from this unfortunate fifteen-year-old rendered "brain dead" after being struck from behind by a truck while riding her bicycle. Her parents had given consent for her to serve as a multiple organ donor. None of the organ programs in the United States had accepted her lungs as satisfactory for anyone in their respective programs and thus the Toronto program had been contacted. We did have a recipient; a young patient with cystic fibrosis whose remaining life was measured in weeks.

Although the Des Moines teenager's lungs seemed to have been damaged by the accident, there was still sufficient doubt as to their utility that a flight to Des Moines seemed worthwhile, especially as this was probably the only chance that the Toronto youngster had. The girl's death would be doubly disturbing for me, as her lungs had deteriorated even further by the time of my arrival and were now beyond the point that I could reasonably consider using them. Thus it was not just her death on my mind but the almost certain demise of the recipient eagerly awaiting my return with the hope that it would signal the promise of new life. I wondered if anyone had yet informed her or her family that the transplant would not take place. Given the scarcity of donors, they would know what that portended.

As I had on so many occasions in the past, I began to second-guess my decision not to take the lungs and give her a chance. Over the years we had begun to accept a degree of donor lung function that in previous years would have seemed irresponsible, and yet we had met with success. Although the function of these lungs seemed beyond any reasonable limit, one always considered that perhaps this was merely the next stage in our development and that all I needed to do was take the chance. But if the chance failed and another donor became available within days, what then . . .

And so the circular argument went about in my brain. It always had. Nonetheless, I anguished for the Toronto family and wondered how I would handle the situation if it were one of my children facing this dilemma. The thought was not new; I had been through this experience several times before. Today, however, such thoughts were not to be sublimated. Like most surgeons, I had come to accept the loss of life or the disastrous complication. It was no doubt the natural result of the surgeon's job, a means of handling emotional trauma. We seemed to be able to compartmentalize the trauma away in a secure part of our brain. We simply "dealt with it" each in his/her way. For some surgeons, the compensatory mechanism prevented them from ever showing empathy or compassion to their patients or their families. In others, it lurked on the periphery of their awareness and made them unsure of their decisions and in the end destroyed their professional skill as indecision and inaction gained the upper hand over sound judgment. For most of us, however, the situation was simply sublimated and accepted as part of our daily practice. The memory was always there and would come to the fore in times of despair, concern, or during periods of reflection. The basic principle, however, was that you must never let it get in the way of your work. But for me, on this day, it had a continued personal impact. It would very much get in the way of my work.

On the return flight I was barraged by images of the dynamics of my own family if one of us were to face the certainty of imminent death. Certainly I was besieged with guilt at the thought of leaving my family with so much unfinished from a personal point of view, so much unsaid or undone because I had been too busy, too committed to my job. I could always rationalize my absence from family events and social occasions because duty called. As my wife used to say, "How can I compete with your patients when they need you?" That thought was bad enough, but was nothing compared to the realization that the guilt would be with me daily were it to be one of my loved ones who left the family circle because of trauma or disease. At least the guilt I felt on imagining my own death would be transient. The depression and self-recrimination that would hound me for the rest of my life upon the death of a member of my family was a realization that was both disturbing and for the first time insightful. The vision did not leave me for several days.

A week later, I decided that the time had come for a radical change in my lifestyle. The desire had been there before, but never so persistent. I had come to recognize that my move to Ottawa had been a sorry attempt at change and was not a move for professional gain even though that was the outward appearance.

But now, to make this change meant bridling my ambition for professional success. It meant determining that inner personal success was more important. It was time for me to place my family first. The decision to leave the forefront of medical/surgical practice brought some inner turmoil. Surgeons have a huge ego and are convinced that only they can provide the necessary care for their critically ill patients. Although I would certainly want to deny it, there was no doubt that I experienced real pangs of concern that I was about to deny my societal responsibilities by withdrawing from the arena of managing the critically ill. What impact would my departure have on my current patients and those yet to develop respiratory illness that would have come under my care? What immeasurable impact would it have if the waiting lists were prolonged, if I denied society my insights and skill? Believe it; as egotistical as it sounds, I actually ruminated about this. All my life I had been striving for excellence, to be the very best at everything I undertook, to fulfill my responsibilities to society, and finally to ensure that I was a somebody, that I would be remembered when I passed on. Remembered by whom and in what manner was another question . . .

I wonder now in retrospect if it was again my ambition seeking to re-establish its dominance in my life. One soon realizes that he/she is expendable. Some make greater contributions than others, but a replacement readily steps in to take over the reins, and you are quickly forgotten. There are a rare few who are remembered and whose memory is sufficiently cherished that there are memorials to them in perpetuity. They are few, and in medicine they are remembered with a lectureship in their name. Perhaps that was what I had been striving towards. A memory rather than a living presence with the ones I held most dear.

I remember so well the retirement of my senior partner shortly after I joined the staff of Toronto General Hospital. Norman Delarue had worked tirelessly at the General for over forty years as a resident and staff surgeon. He had made major contributions to the management of tuberculosis and breast cancer. He retired at Christmas time, even though he was supposed to wait until the following summer. He was simply tired, and called me from his vacation in Florida to tell me that he would not return in January and would I please take over his practice. He returned in June and came to the ward to say hello to his friends and acquaintances and to visit the ward that had been so much a part of his life. Upon his arrival, he was greeted by a new ward clerk and a new nurse, both of whom asked who he was and did he wish to visit a particular patient. They had no knowledge of him, of his contributions, nor of his long association with the hospital. It was as if he had never been there.

Although there were others to appear who knew him, his initial experience guaranteed that he would never return. Perhaps he was able to see sufficiently into the very near future and recognize that his time would soon be forgotten. When he died ten years later, the staff had no knowledge of him. Some of us remembered him fondly as a fine fellow, a superb physician and teacher; but no memorial graces his name. His distress that day is a grim reminder of our transient hold on notoriety.

Some things are meant to happen. My wife, Lesley, has always maintained that to be true. Although I have at times been doubtful of her assertions, "coincidence" this time did seem preordained. At the end of my clinic a few weeks after the Des Moines affair, I received a call from an overseas medical recruiter named Helen Ziegler. Her agency had contacted me months previously after my name had been suggested as a candidate for the chief of the surgical department at a hospital in Riyadh, Saudi Arabia. They had wanted to initiate a transplant program in lung disease. Although I had declined that possibility, the recruiter was back with the offer of chairman of surgery at a yet to be opened hospital in Abu Dhabi, the capital of The United Arab Emirates. To put the icing on the cake, it was to be operated by a Canadian Corporation. The change that this offered was indeed major and would be a long way from home. I was confident that Lesley would not be pleased with the restrictive environment for women in the Arab world and I said so.

"But Dr. Todd," Helen explained, "Abu Dhabi is in the UAE. The restrictions are minor. They offer full freedom for expatriate women and there is also religious freedom."

With this comment, my interest was reawakened. Then to further reel me in, she went on, "By the way, you know the CEO, and he would really like to work with you again."

Stunned, I asked "So who is he?"

"Michael O'Keefe," was the quick reply.

I was amazed as the coincidences kept building. Michael had been the chief operating officer during my tenure in Ottawa and had had the same job at Toronto General after I moved back there in 1993. We seemed to be following each other around. In addition, Michael was without doubt the best hospital administrator with whom I had ever had the pleasure of working. Indeed, for most of them "pleasure" would be a misnomer. But in Mike's case it was an accurate description of our working relationship.

"When can I see you?" I replied. The hook was set and had sunk deep. I was in addition swimming towards the boat!

The magnitude of the change were I to accept the position was overwhelming We would have to sell everything we owned and leave our family and friends behind. On the other hand, it became clear that my workload would be a fraction of what I had come to consider as normal. Financially it would be rewarding— no taxes, no overhead. As Mike said when I asked him why he had taken on this endeavour: "Simple, Tom: adventure and greed."

I would add "and the chance to smell the roses and see my wife."

Lesley and I were sufficiently interested in the possibility that we visited Abu Dhabi and saw first hand the magnificent new medical facility. It was a shell and the halls and rooms were empty. They echoed loudly as we were given our tour. We met the interim medical director in charge of recruiting, several people in human resources, and finally the head of the Health Authority for Abu Dhabi. Their enthusiasm and optimism for the institution was infectious and it was made perfectly clear that whatever expense was required to establish a premier tertiary care facility would quickly be met. This attitude was particularly evident during my meeting with his Excellency, the head of the health authority. His office was opulent and he swept into it like something out of Lawrence of Arabia, his flowing and correctly starched *dishdash* and headdress billowing out behind him. After tea was passed he introduced me to his medical consultant, a man who would later become an unerring thorn in my side. But this day that fellow said nothing more than a perfunctory hello and remained silent throughout my discussion with his chief. The latter amazed me with the initial content of our discussion.

"What do you know of Islam, Dr. Todd?" he intoned.

"Not a great deal, I'm afraid. It is one of the three monotheistic religions and recognizes Mohammed as its principal prophet. But unless I am misinformed, it also recognizes Christ as a prophet"

"Aha, you know that," he replied and a smile full of orthodontically adjusted teeth filled his face. "Can you then identify the characters in the painting behind you?" he asked with a mischievous grin.

The painting depicted a woman holding an infant under a palm tree outside a walled city surrounded by desert. Given the last comments, a cretin could have made the appropriate guess.

"Well," I replied, wondering what this had to do with the hospital, "it looks like Mary with the Christ child."

"Exactly!" he replied enthusiastically. "I am proud to have it hang here, for, you see, the monotheistic religions are very closely woven."

I noted that he made no mention of Judaism. Then he went further.

"But why do you Christians celebrate Christ's birthday in December when we know from the Koran that he was born in July?"

This was beginning to sound like a test. Little, however, did he know that he was dealing with a child of the manse.

"December was the time of several ancient pagan festivals that originated in Mesopotamia," I said. "In fact, December was the Roman festival of Mars, so it would be natural for the early Christians to select this time to celebrate Christ's birth." I knew I was right; but did he, I wondered.

"I am pleased that you know this Dr. Todd," he said, and then without a pause launched into the meat of the conversation. "Tell me about the importance of research in medicine. I am told that it is something we should anticipate incorporating into the medical centre."

Obviously, I thought, I had passed the test if we were now into more significant matters. I went on to explain the role of basic science and clinical research, the importance of evidence-based medicine, and the concept of the bench to bedside approach. As I concluded, he turned to his aide and said, "He is right. This is important. Be sure we bring forward ten to twenty million dollars for a research centre next to the hospital."

If I was stunned before I was now completely overwhelmed. Ten to twenty million just like that! And all following a fifteen-minute conversation! This was action, this was progress, and I was smitten with the prospect of unlimited funds to do all that I knew would be necessary to give them a world class facility. I was clearly landed in the boat by this time. Little did I know that a well-constructed act had just taken place for my benefit.

I yet had to deal with my wife's concerns and decided to discuss it all in detail once we boarded the plane homeward. As the plane took off, I was composing my arguments when she turned to me and said, "You know, I think you should take this job." What a companion! We determined to think of all the ramifications before making a final decision.

If, however, I needed any further convincing, there was the meeting with the surgeon-in-chief of Toronto General that occurred shortly after my return from Abu Dhabi. All the division heads were informed that our budgets were to be cut even further in the next year to permit the hospital to stay in the black. To complicate matters, I had just recruited another surgeon with the assurances that sufficient operating time would be found for him. Despite my protestations that our surgical waiting lists were already too long and that our income had fallen in excess of twenty percent over the preceding years, there was no turning back from the hospital's decision. On the way home that evening, I recognized that there would be no turning back for me, either. My decision had been made.

The weeks that followed were both frightening and exciting. It was a whirlwind of preparation. Lesley was a Trojan taking charge of everything—the sale of the house, the sale of the cottage, the cars, the storage of our furniture. Nothing escaped her attention. We came closer together as we dismantled the life we had built for ourselves. Our children were magnificent in their understanding and support even to the point of hosting a party at one of the downtown Toronto hotels. We knew we were blessed as parents.

At the hospital there were efforts by some of my partners to hold a farewell party, but I was uncomfortable as they had been most generous to us when we had left for Ottawa ten years previously. A second extravaganza seemed extreme. The nurses and other staff, however, arranged a fitting farewell on the surgical floor that I had come to think of as my professional home. The people that I knew I would miss were there, and I delighted in their presence and generosity of spirit.

But then it came time, as it always does at these events, to say a few words of thanks and farewell. I have spoken all over the world at medical meetings and fancy myself rather good at it. I had given eulogies for both my father and mother with barely a falter in my voice. Yet as I stood in that classroom, I felt inadequate to the task for the first time in my life. After thanking my friends for the party, my gaze drifted to the far wall where all the pictures of the thoracic trainees were arrayed in order including my own from residency days. I recognized the time that had passed, as my picture was in the top row. Below stretched those of the numerous residents that I had trained.

I was shattered to see the full truth of what was about to happen. This was truly it—the end of the great adventure. I knew that I would never return to this hospital as a physician. I would never do another transplant. My days at the height of the Canadian thoracic pyramid were over. As I began to speak, the words were choked off by emotion and for the first time in my life I couldn't finish no matter how hard I tried. I looked over at

Lesley and she smiled that smile that said she understood and waved away my embarrassment. It took her smile to tell me that the decision was still the correct one and I loved her more than ever for truly understanding my distress.

The adventure was finished, but what a ride it had been. So many memories of success and failure. I had witnessed the senselessness of death; the patients whose courage was beyond my imagination. Some had faltered in their efforts to cope and overcome the emotion of the dreadful moment when sure death stared them in the face. But there were many others whose dignity was never overcome by their grief and despair. I had witnessed the birth and the fulfillment of an idea and was honoured to have played a part in it. I had seen my colleagues display moments of brilliance but also slip unwarily into avarice and malice. What I remember most are the patients; but then that was always the purpose of the exercise.

About the Author

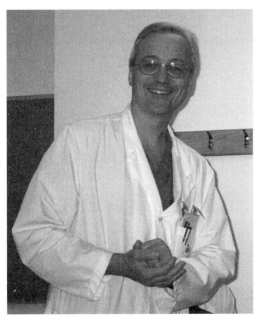

Dr. Todd practised thoracic surgery and critical care medicine at three Ontario Universities—Queen's, University of Toronto, and University of Ottawa. He was the Chairperson of Surgery at the Shaikh Khalifa Medical Centre in Abu Dhabi, the United Arab Emirates. Currently, he is a Senior Medical Officer with the Canadian Medical Protective Association and in his spare time functions as an International Medical Consultant. He and his wife, Lesley, live in Almonte, Ontario, enjoying their four adult children and four grandchildren.

Glossary of Terms

Alveolus Terminal air sacs in the lung where gas exchange with the blood occurs.

Anastomosis The joining of two hollow structures (eg. air tubes, blood vessels) by sutures.

Anticoagulation The use of drugs to prevent the blood from clotting.

Aorta The large artery that delivers oxygen-rich blood from the left cardiac ventricle to the rest of the body.

Asystole No heart action.

Atrium Initial cardiac chamber—one on the left and one on the right side of the heart.

Blood gases A measure of the oxygen, carbon dioxide, and other components in the blood stream.

Bronchus The air tube to each lung after the trachea divides in two.

Bypass	The circulation of blood outside the body through a machine that distributes oxygenated blood, bypassing the heart and lungs. As blood is circulated outside the body through a series of tubes, anticoagulant drugs must be provided.
ECMO	Acronym for extracorporeal membrane oxygenation. A procedure whereby blood is circulated outside the body through a membrane that provides oxygen.
Edema	An abnormal accumulation of body fluid—as seen in swollen ankles or in the lung due to heart failure or trauma.
Endotracheal tube	A tube inserted through the mouth into the trachea to permit the use of a mechanical ventilator.
Etiology	Medical term for the cause of disease.
Fibrillation	Unsynchronized cardiac contraction that leads to a reduction or even disappearance of the circulation.
Graft	Another term for the donor organ.
Hg	Chemical symbol for mercury.
Hypothermia	Abnormally low body temperature.
Idiopathic	An adjective implying that there is no known cause.

Immunosuppression Drug-induced suppression of the normal immune response to infection or a foreign body. Although it prevents rejection of the foreign material (i.e., the transplant), it nonetheless increases the risk of infection.

Inferior vena cava A large vein that drains blood into the heart from the lower body.

Ischemic time The time between extraction of the donor organ and its insertion into the recipient with re-establishment of blood flow.

Omentum Highly vascularized fatty tissue that is in the abdominal cavity.

Oximeter A machine that provides a digital recording of oxygen levels in the blood stream by the use of light transmission through the nail bed via a simple clamp on the fingertip.

Oxygen saturation A measure of the amount of oxygen in the blood stream. Greater than 90% is considered normal.

Pericardium The sac that surrounds the heart.

Pleural space A true cavity referring to the inside of the chest in which the lungs reside. Under normal circumstances, there should not be any attachment (adhesions) between the lungs and the inside of the chest.

Preload The amount of blood returning to the heart. It is high in heart failure and low in hemorrhage or dehydration.

Pulmonary An adjective referring to the lung.

Pulmonologist A term for a specialist in diseases of the lung.

Sinus rhythm The normal contractile sequence of the heart.

Sternum The breastbone.

Superior vena cava The large vein that drains blood to the heart from the upper body.

Suture line The point where two hollow structures are joined together surgically.

Trachea The main breathing tube that one can feel readily in the neck.

Tracheostomy A communication between the skin in the neck and the trachea or breathing tube.

Umbilicus The "belly-button."

Ventilator A machine that forces air into the lungs through either an endotracheal tube or a tracheostomy (see above).

Ventricle   A contractile cardiac chamber that receives blood from the atrium—one on each side of the heart. The right ventricle pumps blood to the lungs; the left ventricle pumps blood to the rest of the body.

To order more copies of

Breathless

by

Thomas R.J. Todd, MD FRCC

Contact:
**GENERAL STORE
PUBLISHING HOUSE**
499 O'Brien Road, Box 415
Renfrew, Ontario Canada K7V 4A6
Telephone: 1-800-465-6072
Fax: (613) 432-7184
www.gsph.com

VISA and MASTERCARD accepted.